Molecular Imaging

Molecular Imaging

An Introduction

Edited by

Hossein Jadvar
Department of Radiology, Keck School of Medicine,
University of Southern California, Los Angeles, CA

Heather Jacene
Department of Radiology, Brigham and Women's Hospital,
Harvard Medical School, Boston, MA

Michael Graham
Department of Radiology, University of Iowa, Iowa City, IA

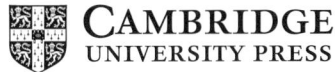
CAMBRIDGE
UNIVERSITY PRESS

CAMBRIDGE
UNIVERSITY PRESS

University Printing House, Cambridge CB2 8BS, United Kingdom

One Liberty Plaza, 20th Floor, New York, NY 10006, USA

477 Williamstown Road, Port Melbourne, VIC 3207, Australia

314–321, 3rd Floor, Plot 3, Splendor Forum, Jasola District Centre, New Delhi – 110025, India

79 Anson Road, #06-04/06, Singapore 079906

Cambridge University Press is part of the University of Cambridge.

It furthers the University's mission by disseminating knowledge in the pursuit of education, learning, and research at the highest international levels of excellence.

www.cambridge.org
Information on this title: www.cambridge.org/9781107621282
DOI: 10.1017/9781107360044

First published 2017

Printed in the United Kingdom by TJ International Ltd. Padstow Cornwall

A catalogue record for this publication is available from the British Library.

ISBN 978-1-107-62128-2 Paperback

Contents

Contributors

Heike Daldrup-Link
Department of Radiology, Stanford University, Stanford, CA

Laura J. Fromme
CellSight Technologies, San Francisco, CA

Daniel Golovko
Department of Radiology, Stanford University, Stanford, CA

Michael Graham
Department of Radiology, University of Iowa, Iowa City, IA

Heather Jacene
Department of Radiology, Brigham and Women's Hospital, Harvard Medical School, Boston, MA

Hossein Jadvar
Department of Radiology, Keck School of Medicine, University of Southern California, Los Angeles, CA

Ramsha Khan
Department of Radiology, Stanford University, Stanford, CA

Andrew Maidment
Department of Radiology, Hospital of the University Pennsylvania, Philadelphia, PA

Amer M. Najjar
University of Texas M.D. Anderson Cancer Center, Houston, TX

Hee Kwon Song
Department of Radiology, Hospital of the University Pennsylvania, Philadelphia, PA

Drew A. Torigian
Department of Radiology, Hospital of the University Pennsylvania, Philadelphia, PA

Shahriar Yaghoubi
CellSight Technologies, San Francisco, CA

Preface

Since the discovery of x-ray by Wilhelm Röntgen at the turn of the twentieth century, there have been monumental strides in the ability to image biological processes in health and in disease. Imaging has not only improved our understanding of the complex and dynamic underpinnings of disease but it has also entered the center of patient care for many conditions. Molecular imaging is a relatively recent term that has been coined in the world of imaging science. The Society of Nuclear Medicine and Molecular Imaging (SNMMI) formed a task force in 2007 to develop standard definitions and terms to serve as the foundation of all communications, advocacy, and education activities in molecular imaging. The task force recommended and the SNMMI board approved the following definition for molecular imaging (1):

> Molecular imaging is the visualization, characterization, and measurement of biological processes at the molecular and cellular levels in humans and other living systems. Molecular imaging typically includes 2- or 3-dimensional imaging as well as quantification over time. The imaging techniques may include radiotracer imaging/nuclear medicine, MR imaging, MR spectroscopy, optical imaging, ultrasound, and others.

The task force further elaborated that

> molecular imaging has relevance for patient care: it reveals the clinical biology of the disease process; it personalizes patient care by characterizing specific disease processes in different individuals; and it is useful in drug discovery and development.

There are a few comprehensive books now available for detailed descriptions of methods and applications in molecular imaging. The aim of this book is to provide a brief introduction to the world of molecular imaging. It is not intended to provide an exhaustive list of all available or potential imaging techniques or methods, but major modalities and applications are included. The book will be useful for students, physicians in training, and others who desire to grasp the basic concepts of molecular imaging in an efficient manner in a relatively short time.

The book is organized by introduction of instrumentation, physics and methods of various imaging modalities, followed by several key biological processes that may be interrogated with molecular imaging. In each chapter, the brief discussion is followed by a bibliography, which may be referred to for additional information and a more in-depth understanding of the topic.

Further Reading

1. Mankoff DA. A definition of molecular imaging. *J Nucl Med* 2007; 48:18N, 21N.

Chapter

1

Instrumentation – CT

Andrew Maidment and Drew A. Torigian

1.1 Introduction to CT

Computed tomography (CT) uses x-rays to generate cross-sectional tomographic images and differs from conventional projection radiography where a snapshot image is taken with a fixed geometry between the x-ray source, the object, and the image receptor. In projection radiography, structures at different depths in the imaged object are superimposed in 2-D, whereas in CT, the 2-D superposition of structures is virtually eliminated. Advanced 3-D-rendered CT images can also be created as needed when contiguous tomographic slices are acquired by a helical acquisition.

CT provides excellent contrast resolution that is far superior to plain-film radiography. However, CT does have inferior spatial resolution relative to plain-film radiography, and does impart substantially more of a radiation dose to patients. Nonetheless, continual advances in CT technology over time have allowed for its practical application in diverse clinical settings, such as with CT colonography, CT angiography, and CT urography for detailed evaluation of colon, vasculature, and urothelial system, respectively.

The CT image is created, in very basic terms, by reconstruction from a large number of *projections*, each of which consists of many *rays* or measurements of x-ray transmission, through a patient. In effect, CT attempts to determine the internal anatomy of the patient by using x-ray projections created at multiple different angles. A typical medical CT scanner is shown in Figure 1.1. In this configuration, the patient lies on the table, and is moved into the opening in the gantry to the desired position. Unseen but inside the gantry are the x-ray tube and detectors, which rotate around the patient. The detectors measure the transmission projections at each of the various angles as the x-ray tube rotates around the patient. After the projections are acquired, a computer is used to reconstruct slices through the patient. The images are then sent to a computer workstation for clinical review.

1.2 Concepts of Attenuation and CT Number

The building blocks for a CT image are a series of transmission measurements of individual rays through the patient, utilizing a thin pencil-like x-ray beam and detectors, as shown in Figure 1.2. The detectors measure the intensity of the transmitted beam, I. The relative transmission is defined as the ratio $-\ln(I/I_0)$, where I_0 is the intensity of the beam entering the patient and is equal to the product of two properties of the patient, the x-ray attenuation coefficient, μ, and the thickness, t.

As shown in Figure 1.2, when x-rays pass through a patient, they are reduced in number or *attenuated*. The x-rays are attenuated via two primary mechanisms. The first of these is *Compton scattering* where the x-ray photon interacts with a free electron and is redirected with reduced energy out of the beam. Such photons are referred to as scattered radiation and are of concern when considering scanner design and image quality. The second attenuation mechanism is the *photoelectric effect*, in which the photon is completely absorbed and thus removed from the beam.

The Compton effect scales with electron density; this results in the Compton effect being nearly independent of the atomic number, Z, of the material. The photoelectric effect, on the other hand, is very strongly dependent on atomic number, where the probability of the photoelectric effect occurring increases proportional to Z^3. Thus, it is the photoelectric effect that is responsible for differentiation between different material or tissue types, when densities are equal. The probability of a Compton effect occurring is almost independent of x-ray energy over the diagnostic range, whereas the probability of a photoelectric effect occurring decreases proportional to the photon

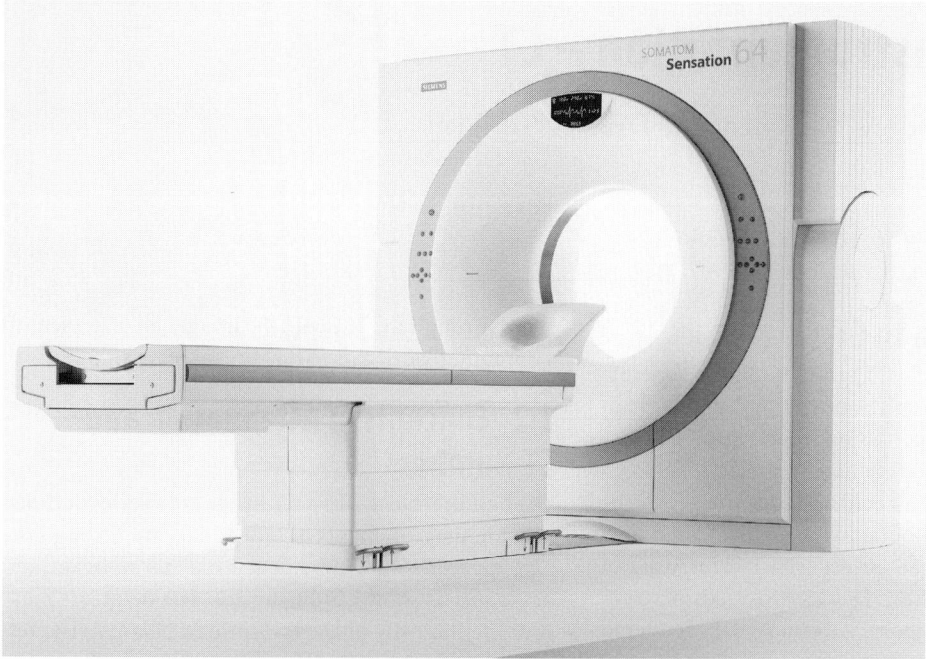

Figure 1.1 A typical CT scanner consisting of a gantry housing the rotating x-ray source and detector arrays. The patient table is moved into the aperture in the gantry for imaging.

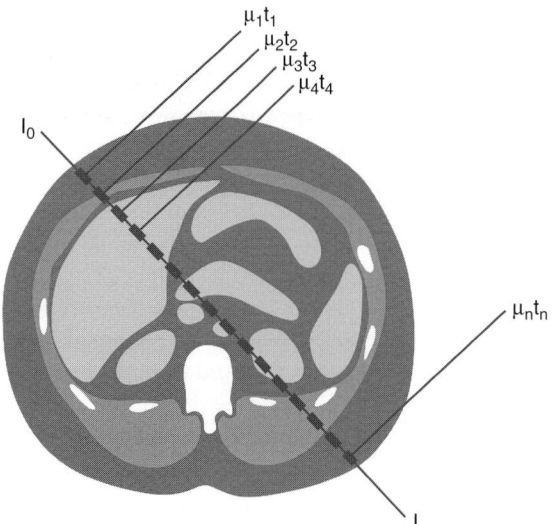

Figure 1.2 X-ray transmission measurements in CT are performed for each ray that passes through the body. The incident x-rays (I_0) are reduced in number after they have passed through the patient (I) due to attenuation by the various tissues of the body ($\mu_n t_n$)

The linear attenuation coefficient, μ, is difficult to work with in practice. A typical result, for example, might be 0.191 cm^{-1} in one region and 0.172 cm^{-1} in a region next to it with good contrast. A quantity called the CT number (in Hounsfield units (HUs)) is therefore used to make more manageable numbers and to reduce their energy dependence by normalizing them to water. The equation relating CT number (in HU) to μ is as follows:

$$\text{CT\_number} = 1000 \frac{\mu_x - \mu_{H_2O}}{\mu_{H_2O}}$$

where μ_x is the linear attenuation coefficient of the voxel of interest, and μ_{H_2O} is the linear attenuation coefficient of water. A difference in CT number of 1 HU corresponds to a difference of 0.1 percent in contrast. The CT numbers for the attenuation coefficients mentioned earlier, 0.191 and 0.172 cm^{-1}, are 0 HU and −99 HU, respectively, roughly the difference between water and fat.

Normalization to water is useful since the body is principally composed of water and is in the middle of the range of CT numbers typical for a scan of a patient (see Table 1.1). It also reduces much of

energy cubed. Thus, the Compton effect dominates for high-energy CT scans and the photoelectric effect dominates at low energy.

Table 1.1 Approximate CT Number Ranges of Human Tissues

Material/Tissue	CT number ranges (in HU)
Bone/calcification/metal/concentrated iodinated contrast material	> 150
Acute hemorrhage	50–90
Soft tissue	20–80
Water	0
Fat	−20 to −150
Lung	−400 to −1000
Air	−1000

the dependence on beam energy. However, atomic composition differences of materials can cause some variation in this rule. Thus, while these differences can usually be ignored over the energy range used in CT, some materials such as iodinated contrast agents are substantially better visualized at lower energies because of the energy dependence of their attenuation properties.

1.3 Principles of CT Image Acquisition, and Helical CT

In all modern scanners, many *rays* are acquired simultaneously, using a *fan beam* configuration as shown in Figure 1.3. A fan beam is a wide, wedge-shaped beam that is thin in the direction perpendicular to the slice (typically called the z direction). A *projection* is composed of the set of rays in the fan beam. An *axial slice* is reconstructed using a series of projections that encircle the patient or object of interest. Thus, the number of transmission measurements required to reconstruct a single slice is given by the number of rays in a single projection multiplied by the number of projections used in the slice.

All modern CT scanners use *slip ring* technology, that is, sliding electrical contacts, to power the x-ray acquisition system continuously, as opposed to older systems that were physically connected by wires, limiting image acquisition to single axial slices at a time. The advent of slip ring technology in the 1990s led to a new method of acquisition called helical (or spiral) CT. In helical acquisition mode, the table moves continuously through the gantry while the x-ray tube rotates around the table, and x-ray transmission data are collected. This continues until the total volume of interest in the patient has been scanned. No delays

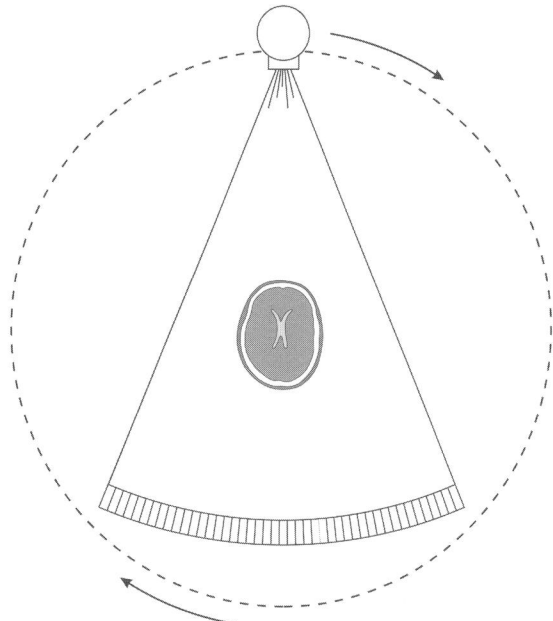

Figure 1.3 Fan beam image acquisition geometry in CT.

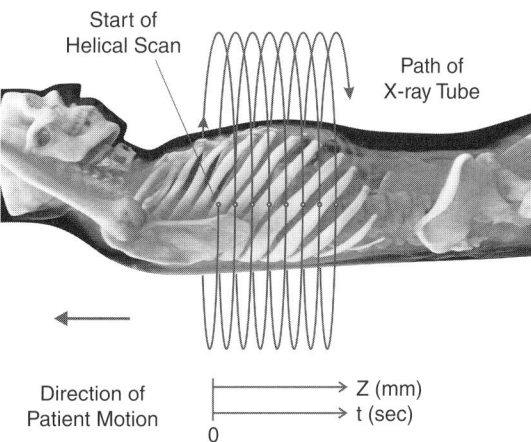

Figure 1.4 Illustration of the helical trajectory of the x-ray tube and detectors around a patient used in helical CT.

between "slices" are required. Tube heating capacity or the ability of a patient to breath-hold may impose some limits on the total acquisition time, however. This helical approach to data acquisition is volumetric, as the data are continuously collected over a volume of tissue, in contradistinction to the axial CT acquisition approach of obtaining single slices one at a time. Figure 1.4 demonstrates the helical trajectory that the x-ray beam makes around a patient in the volume acquisition mode.

Generally, the operator does not directly control the table motion when setting up a helical acquisition. A new parameter is introduced that the operator does adjust in this type of scanning that relates to the tightness of the helix. This parameter is called the pitch and is defined as the amount of table movement per 360° rotation of the x-ray tube divided by the collimator width. For example, if the collimators are set for a 5 mm slice and the pitch is 1.5, the resulting table movement will be 7.5 mm per rotation.

If the data from a 360° segment of a helical CT scan are reconstructed directly without modification, the resulting image will have major artifacts since the patient is undergoing movement by the table throughout the duration of the helical CT scan. It is thus necessary to compensate for this motion by first constructing quasi-planar datasets from the volumetric dataset. The image may then be reconstructed with the standard method that is used for slice-by-slice acquisitions. The construction of quasi-planar datasets is called z interpolation, since the axis along the gantry is the z axis and the tomographic planes are typically constructed perpendicular to this axis.

The most conceptually straightforward z interpolation method is the 360° linear interpolation (360° LI). For a desired slice position z, the projection, $P_z(\alpha)$, at a particular angle α is constructed from the two projections nearest z at the same angle α. One projection will be from a position slightly less than z, $P_j(\alpha)$, and the other will be from one slightly greater than z, $P_{j+1}(\alpha)$. $P_z(\alpha)$ is then constructed from these two projections according to the formula:

$$P_z(\alpha) = (1-w)P_j(\alpha) + wP_{j+1}(\alpha)$$

where w is a weighting factor that is linearly proportional to the relative distance between z and z_j, the z position where $P_j(\alpha)$ was acquired.

While 360° LI is capable of creating high-quality axial images, the resolution in the z direction is degraded. Other z interpolation methods are therefore used which take advantage of the observation that opposing projections essentially demonstrate the same features. In this way, it is possible to construct another (virtual) helix by shifting the original one by 180°. The original and 180° shifted helices can then be used to perform the z interpolation. This interpolation (180° LI) has better resolution in the z direction. Altogether, there are numerous alternative z interpolation methods that can also be employed.

1.4 Multislice CT and Dual-Energy CT

The benefits of helical acquisition are complemented by the recent development of multislice CT (MSCT) (or multidetector row CT (MDCT)) technology. While it is possible to perform multislice axial CT acquisitions, the primary use is in helical CT acquisition. The key component of MSCT is the detector array, which has several rows of detector elements that extend in the z direction, allowing for the acquisition of multiple simultaneous channels of data per gantry rotation (Figure 1.5). The width of a detector element in the z direction depends, in general, on the particular row within which it is located. Different vendors use different combinations of detector element widths of different rows to allow one to acquire varied numbers of slices and slice thicknesses as needed. At present, CT scanners with up to 320 channels of data acquisition are commercially available.

MSCT offers many advantages to single slice CT (SSCT). Scans can be completed more quickly, thus minimizing or eliminating many motion artifacts that occur due to bulk patient motion or from physiological organ motion due to respiration, cardiac motion, or bowel peristalsis, and allow for greater z axis coverage of bodily regions of interest during a CT examination. This gain in image acquisition speed and z axis coverage is particularly important for patients who are not able to hold breath for sufficiently long periods of time, and for patients who are potentially clinically unstable such as in the clinical setting of acute traumatic injury. The quicker scan times also make it possible to perform multiphase CT examinations more efficiently following the intravenous administration of contrast material such as with triple phase liver CT (where noncontrast, arterial phase postcontrast, and venous phase postcontrast images are obtained), 4-D cardiac CT, CT angiography (CTA), and CT urography (CTU). Furthermore, MSCT allows one to obtain scans with a submillimeter section thickness, providing high-resolution images that are isotropic, that is, composed of voxels that are cubic in shape. This minimizes the importance of patient positioning; obviates the need to obtain axial, coronal, and sagittal planes directly, as such images can be retrospectively reconstructed from previously acquired datasets; optimizes CT image postprocessing techniques (discussed in further sections) that can be useful for visualization and interpretation of the image data; and improves quantitative measurement of lesion volumes.

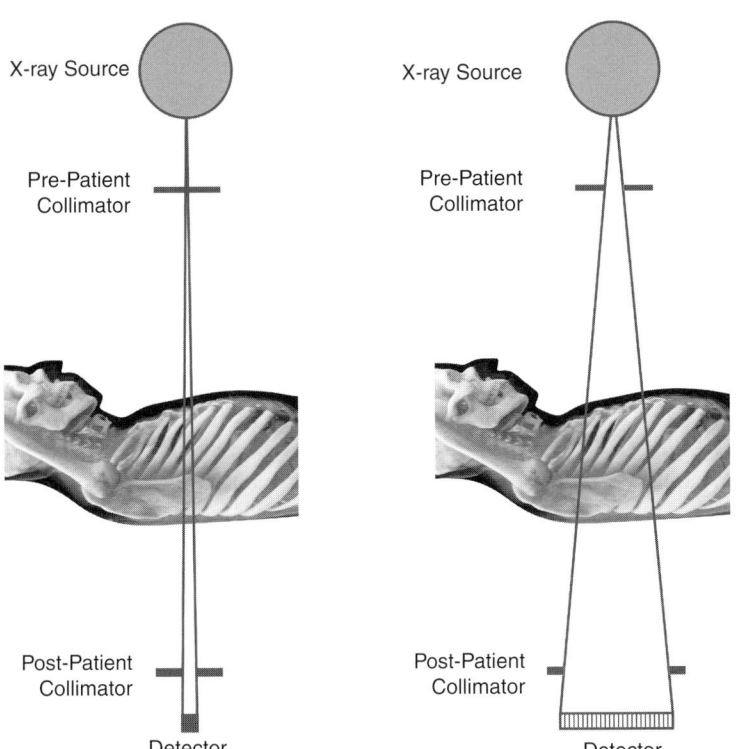

Figure 1.5 Single slice CT (SSCT) scanners (a) have a single row of detector elements, whereas multislice CT (MSCT) scanners (b) have multiple rows of detector elements that extend in the z direction. Note greater z axis coverage by x-ray beam in MSCT scanners compared to SSCT scanners. Also note two sets of collimators; the pre-patient collimator ensures that the x-ray beam striking the patient is as small as possible, while the post-patient collimator defines the width of the beam incident upon the detector, and eliminates scatter.

Another advance in CT technology is dual-energy CT (DECT), which is performed by simultaneously operating the two x-ray tubes of a dual-source CT scanner at different voltage levels (e.g., 80 kV and 140 kV) during patient imaging. Data obtained by DECT may be useful to provide functional information regarding the tissue composition of structures, based on the differential attenuation of the two separate x-ray beam spectra by different tissue components (e.g., calcium, iodine, soft tissue, water, and fat). Such information may potentially be useful for improved lesion characterization, improved quantification of contrast enhancement, and assessment of the chemical composition of renal calculi.

1.5 CT Hardware Components

A CT gantry is shown in Figure 1.1. The aperture of the gantry is the round space through which the patient passes to undergo CT imaging. The patient table, or couch, provides the physical support for the patient and must be strong enough to support overweight or obese patients, yet have sufficiently low attenuation properties so that it does not interfere with the imaging. The table must also be able to move in both vertical and horizontal directions. Movement

in the vertical direction is designed to allow patients to access the table easily, yet ensure that the anatomical region of interest is centered in the gantry aperture for imaging. Movement in the horizontal (z axis) direction is necessary to image the desired region of the patient in either axial or helical modes.

The x-ray system (within the CT gantry) consists of an x-ray generator, x-ray tube, collimators, filters, a detector assembly, and associated electronics. The x-ray generator is responsible for supplying the correct power to the x-ray tube. Virtually all CT generators are of the high-frequency type, as high-frequency generators are more compact than other types of generators, allowing for placement inside of the rotating assembly instead of outside as was necessary with older CT systems. This was another key technical innovation in the 1990s that enabled the development of helical CT.

The production of x-rays occurs in the x-ray tube. The voltage potential provided from the x-ray generator, typically between 80 and 140 peak kilovoltage (kVp), is applied across the tube. The anode is made of a tungsten alloy that is chosen for its relatively high atomic number and high melting temperature, resulting in high x-ray output. The z-flying focal spot (zFFS) technology, available in some CT scanner models, allows for controlled motion of the x-ray tube focal spot in the z direction, leading to a doubling of the number of simultaneously acquired slices in MSCT with further improvement in longitudinal spatial resolution.

The x-rays produced in the x-ray tube are filtered before irradiating the patient. Filtration preferentially attenuates the lower energy x-rays present in the beam since the attenuation coefficient decreases with increasing energy. Filtration is necessary for several reasons. First, a harder, more penetrating beam is desired for CT to reduce patient radiation dose. Second, increased filtration results in an x-ray beam that more closely approximates a mono-energetic source, reducing certain artifacts. However, this must be balanced with the needs of tube loading and of obtaining sufficient x-ray fluence. Finally, additional filtration is provided for beam shaping. This last filter is often referred to as a "bow-tie" filter since it is shaped somewhat in the shape of a bow-tie, where the filter is thinner in the center and is increasingly thicker toward the periphery. This design is used to compensate for the typical ovoid cross-section of the patient, where total x-ray attenuation by the patient's body will be less at the periphery than at the center.

After filtration, the useful x-ray beam is shaped by collimators. These serve to define the size of the x-ray beam. In one dimension, they determine the size of the fan beam. In the other dimension, they determine the slice thickness of the beam. There are normally two sets of collimators, prepatient and postpatient (or pre-detector) (Figure 1.5). The prepatient collimators are physically attached to the x-ray tube and rotate with it, whereas the postpatient collimators are fixed in a position relative to the detectors, and serve to sharpen the profile further. These also absorb much of the scatter radiation produced in the patient/object undergoing imaging, preventing scatter from reaching the detectors and degrading image quality.

After passing through the postpatient collimators, the x-rays are incident upon the detectors. The detector is responsible for converting the x-rays into an electrical signal. It is important that CT detectors have the following characteristics: high efficiency, quick response time, stability, high reproducibility, and large dynamic range. High efficiency assures that most of the useful x-rays contribute to the CT image. This helps to minimize patient radiation dose and image noise. A quick response time is necessary so that afterglow, or residual signal after detection, is minimized, since afterglow can lead to the degradation of spatial resolution. Stability and high reproducibility of detector response are critical since the reconstruction process hinges on the comparison of x-ray intensity with and without the attenuating medium. Detector instability will lead to false readings and the need for more frequent calibrations. The large variations in x-ray intensity seen by the detector make a large dynamic range essential.

The data acquisition system is responsible for taking the analog signal from the detector, converting it to digital format, and sending it to the CT system computer. The computer is responsible for performing the image processing after receiving the data from the data acquisition system. As the data is received, it undergoes preprocessing which includes such tasks as normalization based on the detector calibration. This is then followed by image reconstruction.

1.6 CT Image Reconstruction

After the x-ray data have been collected, they are reconstructed to form an image of the patient or object that was scanned. The raw projection data would produce severe artifacts if reconstructed as is. Therefore, the projection data must first undergo some preprocessing operations before the reconstruction process begins. The first preprocessing step is to normalize the measured intensity to the assumed nonattenuated intensity. The specifics of how this is handled depend upon the scanner design. Preprocessing corrections must also be made since attenuation is not truly linearly related to path length as expected in the ideal case. Scattered radiation, nonlinear detector response, and beam hardening effects all contribute to this.

Filtered backprojection (FBP) is the most common reconstruction method currently in use. In FBP, the projections are filtered prior to undergoing backprojection. The applied filter is designed to remove the intrinsic blurring arising from the backprojection process. Filtering causes a negative shadow to occur on both sides of the backprojected objects. These negative backprojections, when added together for all projections encircling the scanned object, cancel out the false positive contributions caused by blurring.

The operator of the scanner generally has the option of choosing from several reconstruction filters (also called kernels). These filters differ slightly in the

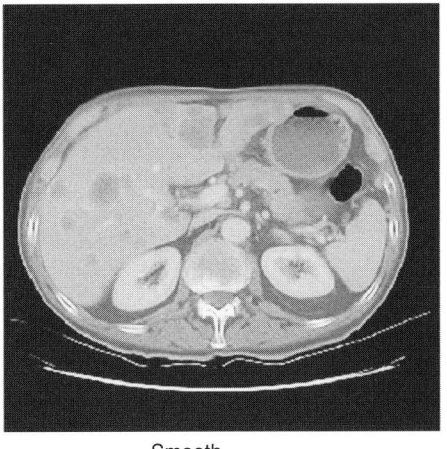
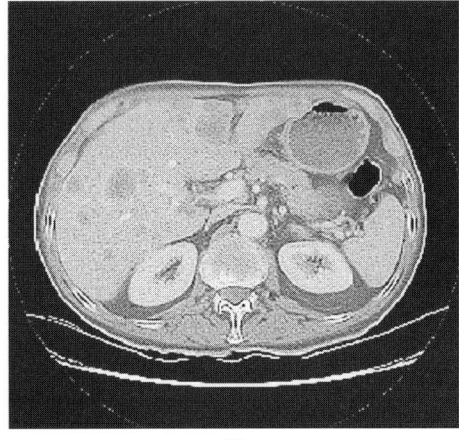

Smooth   Sharp

Figure 1.6 Effect of reconstruction filter (kernel) on CT image quality.

shape of the function used in the filtering process, which in turn influences image quality (Figure 1.6). For example, one filter might enhance spatial resolution at the expense of increasing image noise, whereas another might suppress noise at the cost of decreasing spatial resolution. The filter selected will depend on the information desired. For example, if one desires to detect low-contrast lesions in a patient, a "smoothing" or "soft tissue" filter might be selected since low-contrast lesion detectability is improved given the presence of less noise.

Iterative methods of image reconstruction are beginning to become more popular based on the availability of increasingly powerful computers. In iterative methods, an initial reconstruction of the patient is created. Simulated projections through this reconstruction are then compared to the actual projections. The differences between those projections are determined and used to make a revised estimate of the voxel values. This process is repeated until the differences become sufficiently small as to not further influence the reconstruction. Iterative methods have the advantage that the physics of image acquisition can be modeled, so as to allow for noise reduction or radiation dose reduction.

1.7 Advanced CT Image Post Processing and Display Techniques

In some cases, axial slices are not sufficient to display the imaging features of lesions of interest. In those instances, multiplanar reconstruction (MPR) can be used to improve the depiction of such features. It is possible to display sagittal, y-z plane, or coronal, x-z plane, images rather than traditional axial, x-y plane, images. Oblique planes of section may also be created as needed given the volumetric nature of the x-ray dataset. In fact, MPR images do not even have to be flat, but instead may be curved to follow a particular anatomical structure or lesion of interest. Furthermore, slice thickness may be adjusted accordingly as needed.

The data can also be displayed with volume rendering (VR) (Figure 1.7). This technique uses all of the data in the dataset rather than a subset of the dataset in a given plane or intensity range. Before VR can begin, the data are first preprocessed. Each voxel is assigned a brightness level or color and a transparency level based on its CT number. The image is then built by simulating rays passing through the dataset. The viewpoint is often external to the patient, although it can also be inside the patient. This display technique is useful for purposes of CT virtual endoscopy, where the viewpoint is located from inside the lumen of a vessel, bowel loop, or airway of interest.

Another display technique, which is commonly used in CT angiography applications, is called maximum intensity projection (MIP) (Figure 1.7). In this method, a ray passes through the volume data as it does in other volume-rendering methods. The corresponding pixel is assigned a value equal to the value of the maximum voxel along the ray. This technique has the advantage of preserving the attenuation information in the data, and produces high-contrast images.

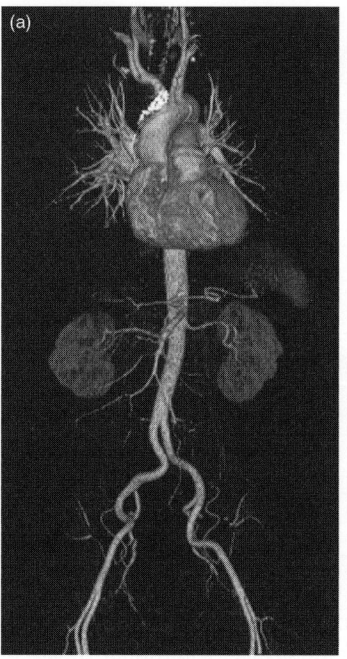
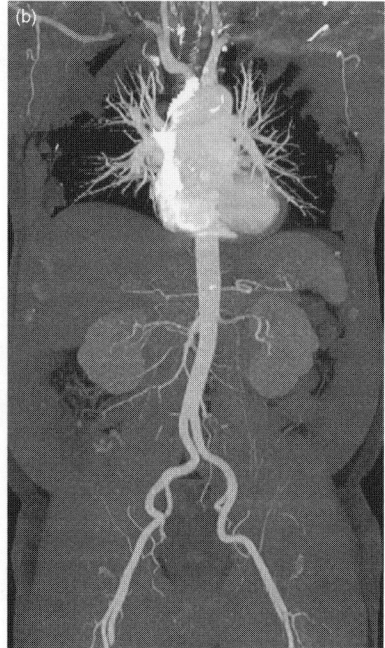
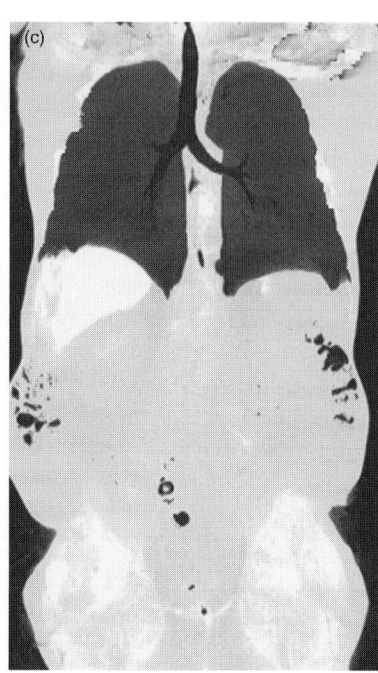

Figure 1.7 Volume rendering (VR) (left), maximal intensity projection (MIP) (middle), and minimal intensity projection (MinIP) (right) display techniques are demonstrated through use of a CT angiography dataset.

One other display technique is called minimal intensity projection (MinIP) (Figure 1.7), where the corresponding pixel is assigned a value equal to the value of the minimum voxel along the ray. This technique may be useful to display lesions involving air-filled structures such as the tracheobronchial tree, lungs, and bowel to best advantage.

1.8 CT Image Quality and Radiation Dose

Spatial resolution is one of the key parameters used to describe image quality. It is a measure of how sharp, or conversely how blurred, the image is. The better the spatial resolution, the closer small high-contrast objects can be placed next to each other and still be discerned as separate entities. The limiting spatial resolution is related to the size of the smallest objects that can just barely be visualized, and is usually quoted in terms of line pairs per centimeter (lp/cm). Typical values for axial CT are around 12 lp/cm. As previously mentioned, the filter used is chosen in part based on its resolution properties.

Spatial resolution in the z axis direction, perpendicular to the tomographic plane, is primarily determined by the detector element size, pitch, and z interpolation algorithm. Smaller detectors or a smaller pitch result in better resolution. The z interpolation method takes data from a region and generates new data to reconstruct a slice at the center of that region. In very general terms, the larger the region used, the broader the sensitivity profile becomes and the worse the spatial resolution is. For example, a 360° algorithm has poorer resolution than a 180° algorithm.

Noise on the images is manifest as random variations of signal in otherwise uniform regions of the patient. The noise in the image limits the ability to visualize low-contrast objects and is measured by determining the number of x-rays used to create a single slice of the patient. Thus, the x-ray acquisition parameters (such as tube voltage, tube current, and exposure time), gantry rotation time, pitch, slice thickness, imaging field of view, image matrix (typically 512×512), z interpolation method, and reconstruction algorithm affect image noise, as well as spatial resolution and radiation dose levels. For example, a decrease in tube current alone will increase noise and decrease radiation dose without affecting the image contrast or CT numbers, whereas a decrease in tube voltage alone increases noise and decreases radiation dose while altering CT numbers and improving image contrast. In general, there is a trade-off between spatial resolution and noise, where improvements in resolution come at the cost of increased noise.

The radiation dose to the patient that is necessary to produce a given noise level will depend on the design of the scanner. Of the parameters that the operator of the CT scanner normally controls, tube current (in milliamperes (mA)) and exposure time (in seconds (s)) are two important ones that affect dose, as radiation dose is linearly dependent on each of these two parameters. Radiation dose also depends on kVp since the number of photons produced changes in proportion to the square of the change in kVp.

The dosimetric quantities used in CT can be divided into doses to standard physical test objects (called phantoms) and patient doses. At the present time, the doses measured from physical phantom studies are used to infer patient doses. However, this practice is under review, and improved patient dose estimation methods are undergoing research evaluation.

The radiation dose to standard phantoms is measured in terms of the CT dose index ($CTDI_{100}$). The $CTDI_{100}$ is typically measured at the surface and the center of the CT dose phantom under axial scanning conditions. These dose values are combined to create an estimate of the dose averaged over the phantom cross-section.

$$CTDI_w = (1/3)*CTDI_{100}(center) + (2/3)*CTDI_{100}(surface)$$

To estimate the dose under a helical acquisition, the dose over the volume of the phantom is calculated as

$$CTDI_{vol} = CTDI_w/Pitch$$

The CTDI is indicative of the dose of a slice through the phantom, typically in units of milligray (mGy). To calculate the dose of a CT procedure, it is necessary to know both the dose per slice and the number of slices acquired. This is quantified by the *dose length product* (DLP), which is calculated as the product of the $CTDI_{vol}$ and the length of the scan, l.

$$DLP = CTDI_{vol}*l$$

The DLP is typically in units of mGy•cm. A typical $CTDI_{vol}$ is in the range of 10–20 mGy. For a 30 cm scan, the DLP would then be 300–600 mGy•cm.

A gross estimate of the effective dose, E, to patients, typically given in units of millisieverts (mSv), can be calculated from the DLP with knowledge of the body parts scanned.

$$E = DLP * k$$

where k is given in Table 1.2. The effective dose is a summary measure of the risk of inducing cancer from the radiation dose of the CT scan. Calculated as described here, this is the effective dose to the standard phantom based on the clinical technique. The actual effective dose to a patient is dependent upon the actual size and age of the patient. Patient dosimetry is an active area of research at the current time, and more representative patient dose measures are anticipated.

Table 1.3 lists the typical effective radiation doses for common CT scan procedures. For comparison, the average background radiation dose for the United States is also provided. The radiation dose from a typical CT scan is comparable to the background radiation dose obtained over the course of one to three years. However, in any discussion of radiation dose, one must generally compare the risks of exposure to the radiation dose to the benefits of the potentially clinically useful diagnostic information that may be obtained from CT. Careful selection of patients to be imaged with CT should be a priority of the radiologist and referring physician in order to avoid unnecessary radiation dose exposure.

Minimization of radiation dose during CT scanning of patients is encouraged, and may be achieved in various ways. Decreases in tube voltage, current, or exposure time, and increases in pitch may be useful

Table 1.2 Conversion Factors between DLP and Effective Dose

Scan location	K
Head	0.0023
Chest	0.017
Body	0.015
Abdomen-Pelvis	0.017
Pelvis	0.019

Table 1.3 Common CT Scan Effective Radiation Doses

Average US background radiation	~3–3.6 mSv / yr
Head CT	1–2 mSv
Chest CT	5–7 mSv
Abdomen CT	5–7 mSv
Pelvis CT	3–4 mSv
Abdominopelvic CT	8–11 mSv
Low-dose chest CT	1–2 mSv

approaches to decrease CT radiation dose while maintaining image quality. Automatic tube current modulation (also called automatic exposure control (AEC)), which automatically modulates tube current in both angular and longitudinal directions in response to the size and attenuation characteristics of the body parts scanned, can also be useful to reduce patient dose exposure by 20–60 percent while maintaining predefined image noise or image quality characteristics. Organ-based tube current modulation (TCM), in which tube current is decreased as the x-ray tube passes over the anterior surface of the body and increased over the posterior surface of the body, may also be used to decrease dose to anterior superficial radiosensitive organs such as the breast, thyroid gland,

and eye lens by up to 50 percent without compromising image quality. Newer reconstruction techniques, such as adaptive statistical iterative reconstruction (ASIR) and model-based iterative reconstruction (MBIR), have shown promise to reduce dose. Through use of ASIR, CT dose can potentially be reduced by up to 65 percent in adults without compromising image quality. Similarly, model-based iterative reconstruction (MBIR) can allow for up to 80 percent reduction of CT dose, although the prolonged processing time may limit its routine use in clinical practice. Finally, use of alternative nonionizing radiation imaging technologies such as ultrasonography (US) and magnetic resonance imaging (MRI) can reduce radiation dose exposure to patients.

Chapter 2

MRI/MRS Instrumentation and Physics

Hee Kwon Song and Drew A. Torigian

2.1 Magnetic Resonance Fundamentals

Magnetic resonance imaging (MRI) involves acquiring signals generated by the protons of water and fat molecules in the body in a strong magnetic field. When an object is placed in an MR scanner, the protons, or spins, will align either parallel or anti-parallel to the field, with a small net number of protons aligning parallel to the field (longitudinal direction), creating a stable equilibrium net magnetization pointing along the main field. When a radiofrequency (RF) wave is applied to the spins, a process referred to as "excitation," the protons absorb the RF energy such that the magnetization is effectively rotated into the transverse plane. This absorbed energy is subsequently released as magnetization returns to its initial state, similar to how a compass needle returns to its preferred equilibrium position (pointing north) when briefly perturbed by a nearby magnet. While the magnetization is in the transverse plane, it precesses about the direction of the main magnetic field, just as a spinning top precesses about the direction of the gravitational field. The frequency with which it precesses is called the Larmor frequency, which is dependent on the strength of the magnetic field and the gyromagnetic ratio, the latter of which for protons is 42.57 MHz/ Tesla. The signal from the precessing magnetization can subsequently be detected using an RF receive coil for purposes of image creation or spectroscopy.

2.2 MR Hardware

A powerful external magnet is a major component of an MR scanner, most commonly with clinically utilized field strengths of 1.5 and 3.0 Tesla, which is placed in a room that is externally shielded by an RF shield to reduce or eliminate interference between radio waves from the outside environment and those obtained from the MRI examination. The high magnetic field strengths are produced by large currents that flow along superconducting wires wound about a cylindrical bore. The superconducting wires are kept cold with liquid helium compartment at ~4° K, which in turn is contained within a second compartment of liquid nitrogen (boiling point ~77° K). In addition, these liquid cryogen compartments are separated from the outermost casing of the scanner by a vacuum layer to minimize heat penetration. As the cryogens slowly boil off over time, they require periodic replenishment.

In order to produce images with minimum artifacts and distortions, the static magnetic field needs to be homogeneous within the imaging field of view. This is achieved with the use of several shim coils which produce additional static magnetic fields to compensate for any field variations that are present, and can be individually adjusted for a particular scan session to achieve the highest level of field homogeneity.

Magnetic field gradient coils are also necessary to create transient linear gradients in the magnetic field in various orientations of interest for purposes of slice selection as well as for frequency and phase encoding of signal positional information in order to create images as described in the chapter.

A transmitter coil is required to send RF excitation pulses, such as through the body coil that is built in as part of the "doughnut" of the machine, whereas local receiver coils are required to receive signals from the tissues of interest. An analog to digital converter is also necessary for converting analog raw data into digital data, which is subsequently processed by a computer to create MR spectra or images.

2.3 T1 and T2 Relaxation Time Constants

Following excitation of the spins into the transverse plane, the rate with which the magnetization returns to the equilibrium position can be described by two time constants, T1 and T2. T1 is the longitudinal or spin-lattice relaxation time constant which describes the time it takes for the magnetization to recover along the longitudinal direction. In particular, $M_z(t) = M_o * (1 - \exp(-t/T1))$, where M_o is the equilibrium magnetization, $M_z(t)$ is the longitudinal magnetization, and t is time following excitation. T2 is the transverse or spin-spin relaxation time constant that describes the time it takes for the transverse component of magnetization to decay. In particular, $M_{xy}(t) = M_o * \exp(-t/T2)$, where $M_{xy}(t)$ is the transverse magnetization at a particular time t. In most tissues, T2 is on the order of 30–100 ms and is typically much shorter than T1 which ranges in 250–2500 ms. Thus, the transverse magnetization usually decays well before full longitudinal magnetization has recovered.

2.4 Image Contrast

One of the greatest advantages of MRI over other imaging modalities is the superior soft-tissue contrast that it can provide. Since different tissues are characterized by different T1 and T2 values, and to lesser degree proton density, one is able to effectively control image contrast by judiciously choosing specific MR timing parameters. For example, to create an image with T1-weighting to highlight differences in T1 among tissues, the time between excitations (or repetition time, TR) could be shortened, which would allow tissues with faster longitudinal magnetization recovery (short T1) to be brighter than those with slower longitudinal magnetization recovery (long T1). To create an image with T2-weighting to highlight differences in T2 among tissues, the time between excitation and signal detection (or echo time, TE), could be prolonged, which would cause tissues with slower transverse magnetization decay (long T2) to be brighter than those with faster transverse

magnetization decay (short T2). Tissues with relatively low proton density, such as lung parenchyma, consistently appear dark in typical MR images. Flip angle is another parameter that can be adjusted to alter T1-weighting, as it determines how much a magnetization is tilted away from its equilibrium position during an excitation. In addition, T1-weighted images can also be obtained after intravenous administration of a contrast agent to improve the detection and characterization of lesions in the body. The typical contrast agent used for this purpose is composed of a gadolinium chelated to an organic compound and provides improved image contrast by predominantly shortening the T1 of adjacent water protons, leading to higher T1-weighted signal intensity of tissues that receive greater levels of blood flow (Figure 2.1).

2.5 Overview of Pulse Sequences

A pulse sequence is an organized set of preprogrammed RF and gradient magnetic pulses used to acquire MR data. There are various types of pulse sequences, including those used to achieve different image contrasts, to selectively image water or fat, or to acquire data rapidly. The simplest of these is the gradient echo sequence, which utilizes magnetic gradients to create a signal called a gradient echo.

This begins with an RF pulse to excite the spins within a desired slice. This is accomplished by simultaneously applying a linear magnetic field gradient perpendicular to the plane of the desired slice. This gradient causes the magnetic field to vary linearly along the gradient direction, causing spins at different positions within this direction to precess at different frequencies in a well-controlled manner. Since a frequency-selective RF pulse can only excite spins which precess within a fixed range of frequencies (its

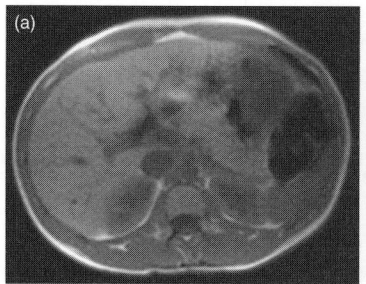 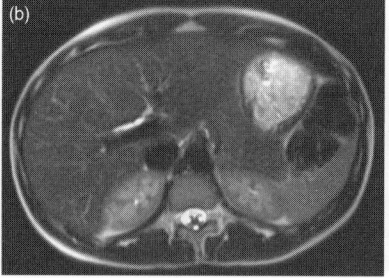 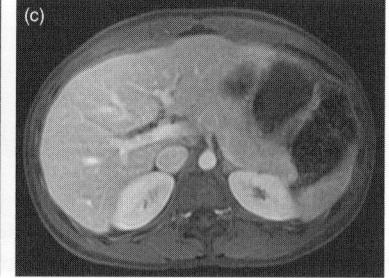

Figure 2.1 The left image is a T1-weighted image, the middle image is a T2-weighted image, and the right image is a contrast-enhanced fat-suppressed T1-weighted image. Note the differential signal intensities of various tissues on these images due to differences in image contrast.

bandwidth), the desired slice thickness can be selected by adjusting the strength of this slice-select gradient whereas the slice location can be selected by adjusting the center frequency of the RF pulse.

In order to obtain spatial information within a selected slice, a second magnetic gradient, the readout or frequency encoding gradient, is applied during the data acquisition period. Similar to the slice-selection gradient, the readout gradient imposes a linearly varying, position-dependent spin precession frequency along the direction of the gradient. This permits the spins at different spatial locations along the readout direction to be distinguished by applying a Fourier transform to the acquired data. In simple terms, just as a glass prism separates white light (which contain all frequencies of the visible spectrum) into individual colors (or frequencies), a Fourier transform separates the combined received signal into individual frequencies, providing spatial information along the readout direction. The number of data points collected during the readout window determines the image matrix size along this gradient direction.

To obtain spatial information within a selected slice in the direction perpendicular to the readout axis, a third magnetic gradient, the phase encoding gradient, is applied prior to the data acquisition period. The amplitude of the phase encoding gradient varies from a maximum positive to a maximum negative value during multiple slice excitations. This permits spins at different spatial locations along the phase encoding direction to be distinguished by differences in their phase. The image matrix size along the phase encoding axis is determined by the number of phase encodings that are applied.

One of the most common uses of the gradient echo sequence is for rapid, T1-weighted imaging applications. With gradient echo imaging, short TRs can be used, on the order of a few milliseconds or less, to obtain images very quickly, often used as the first sequence for localization purposes. The use of a short TR also causes the images to be T1-weighted since the short time between excitations does not allow tissues with long T1s to sufficiently recover their longitudinal magnetizations before the next excitation pulse. Small flip angles (< 30°) of the RF pulses are often used with gradient echo sequences to ensure that sufficient magnetization remains for subsequent excitations.

One of the main drawbacks of the gradient echo sequence is its sensitivity to magnetic field inhomogeneities, either due to an inhomogeneous main

magnetic field or due to susceptibility differences between regions such as at tissue-gas interfaces. These inhomogeneities cause spins within a voxel to precess at different frequencies, resulting in a loss of signal coherence and reducing the voxel intensity. This effect is exacerbated with longer TEs. Since this signal loss occurs while spins precess in the transverse plane, the relaxation time constant is referred to as $T2^*$ (T2-star), comprising intrinsic T2 relaxation effects and magnetic field inhomogeneity effects. Signal loss from $T2^*$ decay is exacerbated at higher field strengths since the susceptibility-related inhomogeneity scales linearly with field strength.

To overcome signal loss caused by magnetic field inhomogeneity, a spin echo sequence can be used. A spin echo sequence is similar to a gradient echo sequence, except that a second RF pulse, the refocusing or 180° pulse, is added between the excitation pulse and data acquisition to create a signal called a spin echo. The main purpose of the refocusing pulse is to reverse the unequal phase accumulation of intra-voxel spins caused by field inhomogeneities. By timing the refocusing RF pulse to occur at time TE/2, exactly in between the excitation pulse and the center of data acquisition, the phase accumulated by spins between excitation and TE/2 is reversed such that it is refocused and becomes zero at time TE. Thus, with spin echo sequences, signal loss will not occur due to field inhomogeneities, but only due to T2 relaxation effects.

2.6 Fast Imaging Sequences

While conventional gradient and spin echo pulse sequences acquire one line of data within each TR, the total scan time can be substantially reduced if multiple lines of data are acquired after each excitation pulse within each TR. In an echo planar imaging sequence (EPI), multiple gradient echoes are acquired following each excitation pulse, significantly reducing total scan time. In single-shot EPI acquisition, the entire set of gradient echoes needed to create an image is acquired after one excitation, although the spatial resolution is typically lower at 64×64 or 128×128. Most functional MRI acquisitions utilize EPI for rapid data acquisition.

Multiple spin echoes can also be acquired in a fast or turbo spin echo (FSE or TSE) sequence, where multiple refocusing pulses are applied, each followed by a data acquisition. In current clinical protocols, the conventional spin echo sequence is no longer used, but instead has been replaced by the FSE sequence, which is typically 16–32 times faster. In single-shot FSE acquisition, the entire set of spin echoes needed to create an image is acquired after one excitation. Both EPI and FSE do have drawbacks, however. EPI images can sometimes have severe distortions in regions close to tissue-gas interfaces due to susceptibility effects, while images acquired with FSE can potentially become blurred due to T2 relaxation, particularly when too many spin echoes are prescribed.

2.7 Dynamic Contrast-Enhanced MRI (DCE-MRI)

Assessment of lesions with intravenous contrast agents can potentially be augmented by observing the dynamic pattern of signal enhancement over time via dynamic contrast-enhanced (DCE-) MRI. Owing to increased vascularity, malignant lesions are typically characterized by greater rates and amounts of early enhancement relative to those of benign lesions. In addition, malignant lesions tend to subsequently washout over time whereas benign lesions often do not. As such, these characteristic enhancement patterns may be useful to characterize lesions as benign or malignant. In addition, by using an appropriate pharmacokinetic compartmental model of contrast distribution in conjunction with signal intensity measurements from tissues of interest and an artery in the field of view (the input function), it is possible to compute various tissue perfusion parameters of interest, such as the volume transfer coefficient between the vascular and extravascular extracellular compartments (K^{trans}). Such parameters may be useful to assess for early response of tumors to anti-angiogenic and anti-vascular therapies during clinical trials.

DCE-MRI, however, often requires rapid imaging techniques to achieve high temporal resolution while maintaining sufficient spatial resolution. Many of the recent developments in MRI technology have addressed this issue, including parallel imaging and alternative image reconstruction strategies.

2.8 Diffusion Weighted Imaging (DWI-MRI)

While the achievable in vivo spatial resolution of MRI is currently on the order of 1 mm^3, it is possible to probe the motion of the water molecules at a much smaller scale via diffusion weighted (DW-) MRI, which utilizes a modified T2-weighted spin echo imaging sequence with diffusion-sensitizing gradients. In particular, following excitation, spins are first "labeled" with the application of one or more gradients, imparting a position-dependent phase to the spins. After a short period of time (~50–100 ms), and following the refocusing pulse which inverts the accumulated phases, identical gradients with the same amplitude and duration are applied to "rephase" the spins. The phase of those spins that are stationary will be completely reversed, so that there is net zero phase accumulation, whereas those of spins that are in motion (e.g., owing to a high diffusion constant) will accumulate a non-zero phase. Tissues with higher diffusion constants will accumulate greater phase. As a result, the total signal from a voxel containing spins that are in motion will be reduced, and moreover, the rate of motion (because of diffusion) along the direction of the applied diffusion gradients will be related to the level of signal loss. Thus, diffusion of water molecules can be observed in tissues and lesions with DW-MRI at a much lower spatial resolution.

DWI-MRI is an effective tool for early detection of acute cerebral infarction, as cellular swelling and cytotoxic edema lead to a restriction in water molecule diffusivity. It is also useful for improved detection and characterization of malignant lesions in the liver and other organs, as well as for early tumor response assessment purposes. Viable tumors are typically cellular, leading to restricted water molecule diffusivity, whereas treated tumors become less cellular, leading to fewer cellular and subcellular compartmental membranes and hence less restricted water molecule diffusivity (Figure 2.2).

2.9 Magnetic Resonance Spectroscopy (MRS)

Magnetic resonance spectroscopy (MRS) is a non-invasive MR method that allows for quantification of the abundance, type, and location of endogenous molecular compounds within tissues of interest. It does so by taking advantage of the quantum-mechanical properties of the nuclei of certain isotopes, which allow them to be manipulated through the use of RF pulses and magnetic fields. MRS is most often based on ^1H given its abundance in tissue, although it can be based upon other nuclei such as ^{13}C, ^{23}Na, or ^{31}P, among others. The signals obtained from one or more voxels of interest sampled within a particular lesion

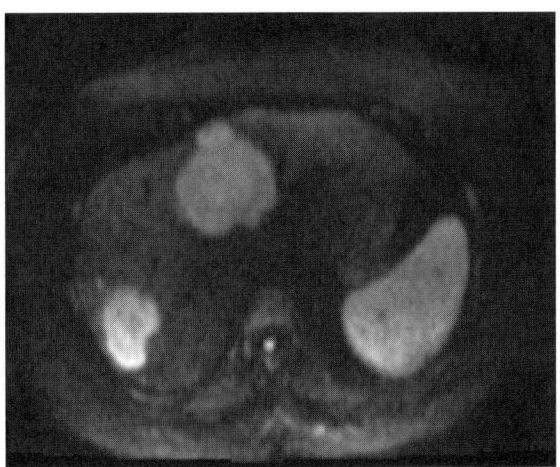

Figure 2.2 Diffusion-weighted image showing multiple liver metastases with high signal intensity due to restricted diffusion.

or tissue are typically displayed as a series of spectral peaks of different chemical compounds of variable amplitude and nuclear precession frequency in relation to those of a reference standard molecule.

MRS has most often been applied clinically to assess brain lesions. However, it is limited by suboptimal sensitivity in the millimolar concentration range, its technical complexity of implementation, lack of standardization across vendors and institutions, and the potential for sampling error if large or multiple lesions of interest are present.

2.10 MR Safety

Since MRI relies on a powerful magnetic field to create images, one of the potential dangers is the possibility of a ferromagnetic object being pulled into the bore of the magnet with enormous force. A 3 Tesla scanner has a field strength that is approximately 5 orders of magnitude stronger than the earth's magnetic field, and is strong enough to attract a floor buffer, a chair, or even a pen into the scanner. However, since the magnetic field falls off rapidly with distance from the bore of the magnet, objects must be in close proximity to be affected by the strong field. To prevent accidental injuries, every patient is carefully screened to ensure that non-MR compatible metallic objects are not taken into the scanner room, and metal detectors are also often utilized for this purpose. Many modern medical devices, such as cardiac pacemakers and stents, are now MR compatible, allowing patients with these appliances to be scanned, although there may still be undesirable image artifacts such as signal loss and image distortions.

A second safety concern is RF heating of the patient during the scans. Since many RF pulses are typically necessary to create MR images, the total power and peak power that are being deposited to the body must be monitored. Federal guidelines have been set to limit the amount of heat that can be delivered to the body during MRI, which is measured by the specific absorption rate (SAR) in units of W/kg. Another safety concern is the rate of change of the magnetic field that can potentially cause nerve stimulation, such that a maximum gradient slew rate has also been set by the FDA. All vendor-approved pulse sequences must meet these federal guidelines prior to use in humans.

Optical and Ultrasound Imaging

Michael Graham and Hossein Jadvar

3.1 Optical Imaging

Optical imaging has been used by countless species since the evolution of the eye. It is used as a critical observational technique in assessing the skin of patients by dermatologists. It is used for internal examination by endoscopists. However, following the invention of the microscope in the late 1500s, optical imaging began to be extended to much smaller objects. The capabilities of the microscope have evolved over the recent centuries, with many different approaches, such that it is impossible to fully review optical microscopy in a brief chapter. The major focus of this chapter is fluorescent and bioluminescent imaging in small animals, and when feasible in humans. A recent textbook that covers the subject area in greater depth is *Biomedical Optical Imaging*. The reader can also find an excellent review of general microscopy in Wikipedia and of optical microscopy at the Olympus Microscopy Research Center.

3.1.1 Fundamental Issues

As photons propagate through tissue, they are attenuated and scattered. The degree of attenuation and scattering depends on the wavelength of the light and the characteristics of the tissue being imaged. In most animals, including humans, a major determinate of the absorption of light is hemoglobin. Visible light extends from 380 nm (deep violet) to 750 nm (dark red). Hemoglobin absorbs markedly from about 500 nm to 600 nm, with significant difference in absorption between oxygenated and deoxygenated hemoglobin. Above 600 nm, extending into the near infrared, the absorption is much less, allowing penetration of photons to several millimeters or even centimeters. This illustrates why near infrared imaging is the favored part of the spectrum to use for in-vivo optical imaging.

3.1.2 Fluorescence Imaging

The essential elements of fluorescence imaging are: (1) existence of a *fluorescent molecule* within tissue that has localized there by bulk flow (i.e. blood vessels or lymphatics), binding to a receptor, or metabolic trapping; (2) *illumination of the tissue* with a light source of appropriate wavelength, which excites the fluorescent molecule; and (3) a *detection system* that can image the emitted light from the fluorescent molecule.

3.1.2.1 Fluorescent Molecules

Most fluorescent molecules are selected to localize preferentially, by binding to a receptor or by metabolism, and have a fluorophore covalently attached. Fluorophores typically are small molecules (200–1000 MW) and contain several combined aromatic groups, although fluorescent proteins are somewhat larger. These include green, yellow, and red fluorescent proteins (GFP, YFP, and RFP respectively).

There are a large number of non-protein fluorophores that can be used to label organic molecules or can be used alone. Two fluorescent molecules that have been approved by the FDA for use in humans are fluorescein and indocyanine green (ICG). Fluorescein is activated by blue or ultraviolet light and has peak emission in the green. It has been used extensively in ophthalmology. Indocyanine green has been used for blood volume, liver function, and liver blood flow studies for years. Generally these studies were done with multiple timed blood sampling and analysis using colorimetry. More recently it has become known that indocyanine green fluoresces in the near infrared with excitation between 760 and 785 nM and emission between 820 and 840 nM. This agent has been used extensively in the visualization of lymphatic vessels in a number of settings.

Although it is convenient that ICG is an approved agent that can be used in humans, there are several other fluorophores that have far brighter fluorescence and are in clinical trial. One of these will likely replace ICG, once it is FDA approved.

3.1.2.2 Tissue Illumination

Excitation has to be at a higher energy than the emission. If filters are used, it may be possible to block the illuminating light and only see the fluorescence. When ultraviolet illumination is used, because of the low sensitivity of the eye to ultraviolet, only fluorescence is seen. For near infrared fluorescent imaging, a laser is frequently used to provide excitation. In some settings, it is useful to focus and scan the laser beam to achieve higher resolution. This has been very successfully used in fluorescent microscopy.

3.1.2.3 Detection Systems

Detection can be as simple as visual observation, if the fluorescence is in the visible part of the spectrum and is sufficiently bright. If it is not, more sensitive detectors are needed. Infrared imaging detectors have been developed for night vision goggles, thermography, meteorology, and astronomy, as well as other nonmedical uses. This means a wide variety of detection systems is available. When the fluorescence is not very bright, or when some degree of quantitation is needed, the imaging is done in a light-tight box.

3.1.3 Bioluminescence Imaging

Bioluminescence imaging is usually used in small animals for preclinical studies. The light that is produced arises from an enzymatic reaction between a luciferase enzyme and its substrate. The most commonly used system is firefly luciferase and the substrate is luciferin. A typical experiment would utilize a tumor cell line that has had the gene for luciferase incorporated into its DNA. The tumor is then implanted into an immune-incompetent host, such as a nude mouse. As the tumor grows or is affected by experimental therapy, it can be visualized by injected luciferin, usually intraperitoneally. The luciferin binds to the luciferase and light is emitted. The light from firefly luciferase is orange-yellow and peaks at about ten minutes after injection. The light level is reasonably stable for about one hour. The animal is then anesthetized and imaged with a very sensitive digital camera in a light-tight box. Specialized imaging systems for this purpose are available from a number of manufacturers, including Brucker, Berthold, Li-Cor, and Perkin-Elmer.

There are several other luciferases available, such as from the click beetle and the sea pansy; however, firefly luciferase is the most widely used.

3.1.4 Photoacoustic Imaging

Photoacoustic and thermoacoustic imaging are hybrid imaging techniques that depend on the expansion of tissue that occurs following delivery of short, focused pulses of energy. With photoacoustic imaging the pulses are delivered from a laser and in the case of thermoacoustic imaging the energy comes from pulsed focused microwaves. In both cases an ultrasonic probe is used to visualize the signal. It has the advantages of lower cost instrumentation, compared to CT or MRI, and better depth capability compared to near infrared frequency. It is used primarily for visualization of anatomic and vascular structures with a spatial resolution of 100–200 μM.

3.2 Ultrasound Imaging

Ultrasound imaging systems use the propagation of ultrasonic (mechanical) waves from a transducer into the tissue and form images based on the resultant detection of the reflected waves (echo) as a consequence of differing acoustic (mechanical) properties of tissue interfaces. The imaging performance of the system depends on the frequency of transmitted waves and the tissue mechanical properties. The fundamental trade-off is the inverse relationship between ultrasound frequency and depth of penetration. Higher frequency results in better resolution but poorer penetration. The use of diagnostic ultrasound is ubiquitous in clinical medicine in view of its ease of use, portability, real-time imaging capability, relatively low cost, and safety. High-resolution ultrasound imaging systems have become available for molecular imaging research employing a number of methods including 2D and 3D imaging, color and power Doppler (suited for imaging blood velocity and perfusion), elastography (tissue stiffness) and use of intravenous non-targeted and targeted microbubble contrast agents (which may be used for diagnosis or delivery of localized therapy). The interested reader is referred to several excellent published reviews on the fundamental basis and application of this molecular imaging technique.

Further Reading

1. Fujimoto JG, Farkas DL, Eds. *Biomedical Optical Imaging*, Oxford University Press, 2009 New York.

2. www.olympusmicro.com/primer/opticalmicroscopy

3. Polom K, Murawa D, Rho YS, Nowaczyk P, Hünerbein M, Murawa P. Current trends and emerging future of indocyanine green usage in surgery and oncology: a literature review. *Cancer*. 2011 Nov 1;117(21):4812–22.

4. Sevick-Muraca EM. Translation of near-infrared fluorescence imaging technologies: emerging clinical applications. *Annu Rev Med*. 2012; 63:217–31.

5. Ntziachristos V, Bremer C, Weissleder R. Fluorescence imaging with near-infrared light: new technological advances that enable in vivo molecular imaging. *Eur Radiol*. 2003 Jan;13(1):195–208.

6. O'Neill K, Lyons SK, Gallagher WM, Curran KM, Byrne AT. Bioluminescent imaging: a critical tool in pre-clinical oncology research. *J Pathol*. 2010 Feb;220(3):317–27.

7. Xia J, Wang LV. Small-animal whole-body photoacoustic tomography: a review. *IEEE Trans Biomed Eng*. 2014 May;61(5):1380–9.

8. Foster FS, Cheung K, Cherin E. Ultrasound. In: Molecular Imaging-Principles and Practice. Weissledder R, Ross BD, Rehemtulla A, Gambhir SS (Eds.). *People's Medical Publishing House*, Shelton, CT, 2010. pp. 225–36.

9. Wen Q, Wan S, Liu Z, Xu S, Wang H, Yang B. Ultrasound contrast agents and ultrasound molecular imaging. *J Nanosci Nanotechnol* 2014; 14:190–209.

10. Hyvelin JM, Tardy I, Arbogast C, Costa M, Emmel P, Helbert A, et al. Use of ultrasound contrast agents in preclinical research: recommendations for small animal imaging. *Invest Radiol* 2013; 48:570–83.

11. Lin Y, Chen ZY, Yang F. Ultrasound-based multimodal molecular imaging and functional ultrasound contrast agents. *Curr Pharm Des* 2013; 19:3342–51.

12. Unnikrishnan S, Kilbanov AL. Microbubbles as ultrasound contrast agents for molecular imaging. Preparation and application. *AJR Am J Roentgenol* 2012; 199:292–9.

13. Kiessling F, Bzyl J, Fokong S, Siepmann M, Schmitz G, Palmowski M. Targeted ultrasound imaging of cancer: an emerging technology on its way to the clinic. *Curr Pharm Des* 2012; 18:2184–99.

Instrumentation-Nuclear Medicine and PET

Michael Graham

4.1 Dose Calibrator

In all clinical and research studies involving injection of radiotracers, it is essential to know the amount of radioactivity injected.

The amount of radioactivity is expressed in Becquerels (Bq), the SI unit, or in Curies, the traditional unit. One Becquerel is equivalent to one disintegration per second of the radioactive material. One Curie is equivalent to the rate of disintegration of one gram of Radium-226, or 3.7×10^{10} disintegrations per second. It is apparent that the Becqueral is a relatively small amount of radioactivity and the Curie is a very large amount. Generally relevant doses in humans or animals are expressed in MegaBecquerals (MBq) or MilliCuries (mCi). One mCi = 37 MBq.

The amount of radioactivity for injection is usually measured in a dose calibrator (Figure 4.1). This device consists of two concentric metal cylinders, insulated from one another, with a dry gas in the middle and 100–300 volts between them. When a radioactive object is placed into the middle cylinder, the high energy photons ionize the gas between the cylinders and a current flows. The current is measured and scaled to display the amount of radioactivity in units of either MBq or mCi (or KBq or μCi). Dose calibrators are very reliable and are linear over a large range of radioactivity, but are not accurate for measuring very small amounts (< 100 kBq).

Dose calibrators are calibrated for accuracy using a long-lived source of known activity, usually Co-57 or Cs-137. They are also usually checked daily for constancy (i.e. they always get the same reading).

4.2 Well Counter

Most well counters consist of a cylinder of sodium iodide with a hole in it, along with a photomultiplier (PMT) tube to detect the light pulses that occur when a high-energy photon is absorbed in the sodium iodide (Figure 4.2). Photon events are counted one by one, so

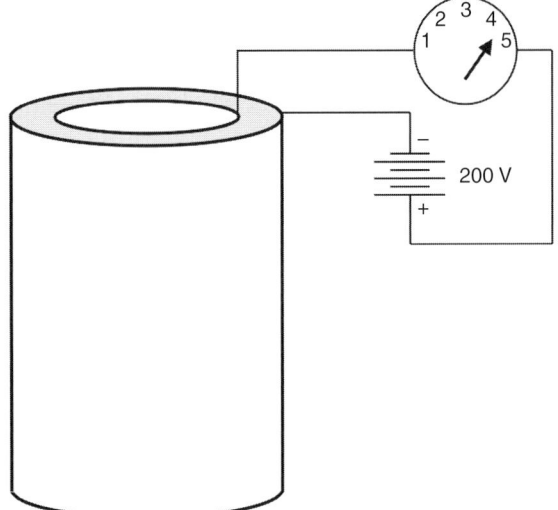

Figure 4.1

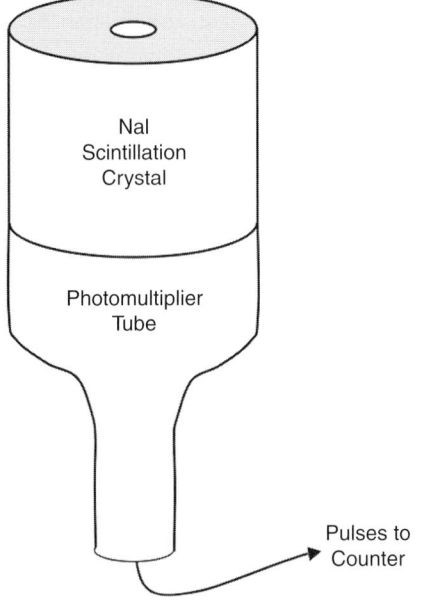

NaI
Scintillation
Crystal

Photomultiplier
Tube

Pulses to
Counter

Figure 4.2

well counters are much more sensitive than dose calibrators. The crystal and PMT are housed in a lead enclosure to minimize detection of extraneous radiation.

Most samples are placed into a test-tube, which is then placed into the well (the hole in the crystal). The counter is capable of accepting pulses only in a specific range of amplitudes, and since the amplitude of the pulse is proportional to the energy of the original high-energy photon, it is possible to count more than one isotope at the same time and avoid counting lower amplitude pulses, which are likely to represent noise or scattered photons. Many well counters have an automated sample handling system that changes the test tubes at predetermined intervals and records the counts.

4.3 Gamma Camera

The gamma camera is the primary tool in nuclear medicine to make images of the distribution of radioactivity in patients (Figure 4.3). The scintillator crystal is made of sodium iodide and is typically about 1 cm thick. When a high energy photon is absorbed by the crystal, a flash of light is emitted. By measuring the amplitude of the light pulses seen by the photomultiplier tubes (PMTs) behind the crystal, it is possible to calculate the location of the light flash within about 3 mm. The signals from the PMTs are digitized, the X-Y location of the event is calculated, along with the amplitude of the flash (Z), and then the data is transmitted to a computer system. The electronics are very fast, and can handle as many as 500,000 events per second.

In front of the crystal is a parallel-hole collimator, essentially a plate of lead with many parallel holes in

it. If a high energy photon is directed perpendicular to the crystal, it will go through a hole and be detected. If it is directed at an angle, then the photon will be absorbed by the lead in the collimator and not be detected. In this way the collimator acts as the lens of the gamma camera and results in the formation of a two dimensional image of the distribution of radioactivity in front of the camera.

The counts in a gamma camera image per cm² are proportional to the amount of activity present in the area imaged; however, more superficial activity results in higher count rate than deeper activity. Because of this attenuation, gamma camera images usually cannot be used to measure absolute activity in-vivo. However, these images are often useful for measuring relative activity, such as right versus left lung or kidney activity.

4.4 Single Photon Emission Computed Tomography (SPECT)

The term "single photon" is used to distinguish this technique from positron tomography, which involves detection of two photons at the same time.

SPECT imaging involves rotating the gamma camera around the subject to obtain views over 360° (Figure 4.4). When these images are played as a cine-loop, the subject appears to rotate. These original, raw images are used to calculate reconstructed transaxial images. Most computer systems are set up to display the transaxial images, along with coronal and sagittal images. A major advantage of SPECT images over planar gamma camera images is that deep structures can be seen better, since they are not obscured by overlying activity.

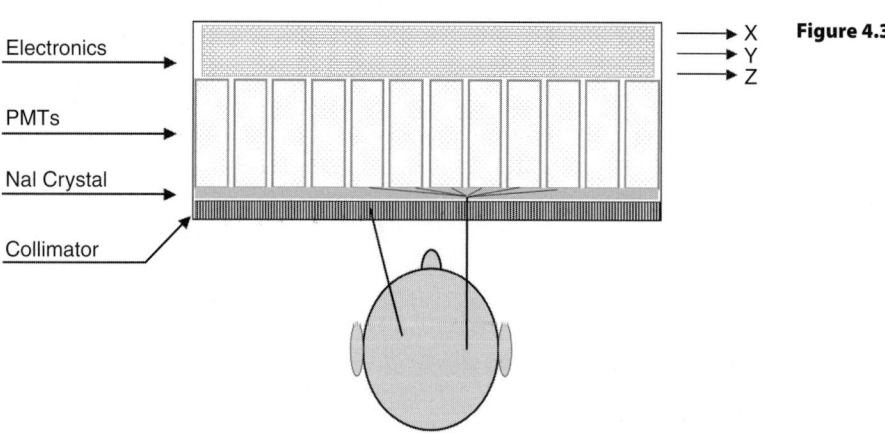

Electronics

PMTs

NaI Crystal

Collimator

X
Y
Z

Figure 4.3

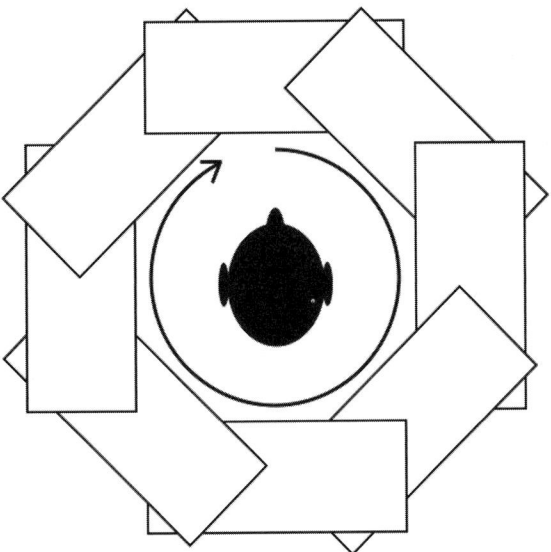

Figure 4.4

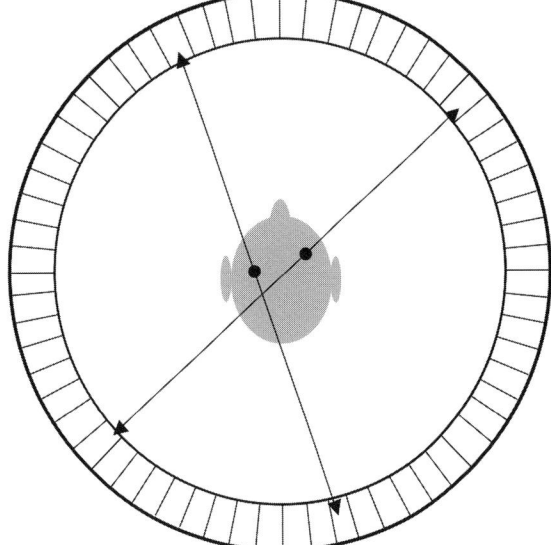

Figure 4.5

Another significant advantage is that counts per ml can be determined as a measure of absolute activity within the subject. Unfortunately the counts per ml may not be accurate because of the necessary corrections that are applied to the data as it is reconstructed. The two major problems are attenuation and scatter. Some of the photons that are emitted by radioactivity within the body are absorbed before they leave the body. The amount of attenuation can be a large factor, up to 10. Scatter is when a photon starts off in one direction, but interacts with the tissue and gets deflected into another direction. It will then appear to come from the wrong part of the body. This is another significant correction that can affect the accuracy of counts/ml from within the body. There are methods to correct for both of these effects, but they are inexact, so quantitative imaging with SPECT is problematic.

4.5 Positron Emission Tomography (PET)

When an atom such as C-11 or F-18 decays, a positron is emitted at high energy and may go for a few mm before it slows down, bumps into an electron, and annihilation occurs. The entire mass of the positron and electron are converted into energy, yielding two 511 KeV photons that are almost exactly directed opposite from each other. The reason that there are two photons is that following annihilation, there is nothing left to take the recoil, and therefore to conserve momentum, there have to be two photons. The positron tomograph is a system designed to detect these annihilation photons (Figure 4.5). The detectors are scintillation crystals with photomultiplier tubes to detect the light output. The crystals are arranged in rings with up to thirty-two adjacent rings of detectors over approximately 16 cm. Although sodium iodide has been used in the past, the current PET systems use other scintillation material, such as bismuth germanate (BGO) or lutetium oxyorthosilicate (LSO).

There are three types of events detected by the tomograph – true, random, and scattered events. True events originate in the subject, do not undergo scattering, and are detected by detectors on opposite sides of the ring within a very narrow timing window, typically six nanoseconds. Random events originate from two different annihilation events that happen at almost the same time. These events can be minimized by narrowing the timing window as much as possible. Scattered events occur when one or both of the photons are deflected as they leave the subject. They can be minimized by not accepting events below an energy threshold level.

As with SPECT, the reconstructed images have to be corrected for both attenuation and scattering. Attenuation correction is more accurate and is usually done using a conventional CT to obtain an attenuation map. Scatter correction is less exact, but overall PET images are more quantitatively accurate than SPECT, and can be used to measure absolute activity in-vivo. These measurements in turn can be used to accurately estimate physiologic parameters of interest such as blood flow, metabolic rates, or receptor densities.

Quantitation-Nuclear Medicine

Michael Graham

5.1 Biodistribution

Perhaps the simplest example of radiotracer quantification is the biodistribution study done in small animals, such as mice or rats. The animal is sacrificed at some well-defined time after administration of radiotracer, various organs are removed, weighed, and then counted in a scintillation well counter. The resultant counts are usually determined in units of counts per minute (cpm) per gram. These counts are meaningful only in comparison to some other count such as the administered dose or in comparison to other tissues, that is ratios. Such ratios are often useful measures of uptake, that is heart:blood, brain:muscle, tumor:muscle, and so on, but are not an adequate description of tracer behavior by themselves. A high tumor:muscle ratio can be due to high tumor uptake or low muscle uptake. Without a measure of absolute uptake, it is not possible to judge if the uptake is high enough to be experimentally or clinically useful. The other problem that is inherent in simple biodistribution studies is that the activity in tissue is dynamic and thus is dependent on the timing of the sacrifice of the animal. The selection of the appropriate time is not trivial and needs to incorporate an understanding of the physiologic behavior of the tracer. Some tracers, such as highly diffusible blood flow tracers (water, butanol, iodoantipyrine), have very rapid kinetics and sacrifice is often within seconds after intravenous administration. Others are taken up more slowly and reach steady state only after hours.

5.2 Indicator Dilution

Plasma and red blood cell volumes are commonly determined using the method of indicator dilution. The underlying concept is that the concentration of an inert tracer in a volume is the amount administered divided by the volume, that is $C = X/V$, where C is the concentration (μCi/ml), X is the amount administered (μCi), and V is volume (ml). Volume can be measured

in another version of the formula: $V = X/C$. For plasma volume determination, plasma concentration is usually measured in a well counter in units of cpm/ml. It is somewhat more complex to determine the amount administered in the appropriate units, that is cpm. The simple approach is to put the injected dose into a well counter just before injection and determine the cpm. This usually does not work because the injected dose is in a small syringe which has very different geometry from the tissue samples which changes the counting efficiency, and because the injected dose often has too much activity to be counted accurately by the well counter. The usual answer to this problem is to make a standard. A standard, in this setting, is a known fraction of the administered dose. Two major approaches are used: (1) When very small volumes are injected, that is 0.1 ml, a volume equal to the injected volume is pipetted and diluted in 100 ml of liquid, typically saline. Then 1.0 ml is counted and multiplied by 100 to yield the injected cpm per ml. (2) When larger volumes are injected, that is 10 ml, the injection syringe is weighed carefully on a laboratory balance (W_0 g), approximately one-tenth of the contents is injected into a partially filled 1 liter volumetric flask, and the syringe is reweighed (W_1 g). Following injection into the subject, the syringe is weighed again (W_2 g). The volumetric flask is filled to the mark, well mixed, and 1 ml is counted (cpm_{std}). The injected dose (cpm_{inj}) is then: $cpm_{inj} = 1000 \, cpm_{std} (W_1 - W_2)/(W_0 - W_1)$.

5.3 Left–Right Comparisons

Clinical planar gamma camera quantitative imaging often involves comparison of the activities in the two lungs or two kidneys. Exact correction for attenuation is not necessary when the goal is to obtain an accurate ratio of activities in the two organs. The usual approach is to obtain anterior and posterior images, determine the counts from the organs, background correct, and combine the anterior and posterior counts by *geometric averaging*, that is the square root of the product of two numbers. Because of the exponential nature of attenuation, geometric averaging is the correct approach.

5.4 Partial Volume Effect

Because of the limited resolution of single photon emission computed tomography (SPECT) and positron emission tomography (PET) images, relatively small objects appear to be less intense than larger objects even when the activity per gram of tissue is the same. If an object is smaller than three times the spatial resolution of a system (in full-width-half maximum – FWHM), there will be some partial volume effect that will reduce the measured activity in an object below its true activity.

Because of partial volume effect, average activity in a region of interest cannot be determined accurately unless the object is relatively large. Exact correction for partial volume is complex because it requires consideration of the size and shape of the hot object, as well as the distribution of regional background activity, and has not become practical yet.

5.5 Planar Attenuation Correction

Attenuation for individual subjects can be measured using a uniform flood source with the same radioisotope as is being imaged. This can be done on a pixel-by-pixel basis and is most conveniently done with a two-headed gamma camera system.

A calibration factor is required to convert the cpm per pixel into $\mu Ci/cm^2$. The most convenient way to do this is to measure the $\mu Ci/ml$ in the flood source. Once the depth of the flood source is determined then the $\mu Ci/cm^2$ can be calculated (see Figure 5.1). The calibration factor (units of cpm per pixel/ $\mu Ci/cm^2$) is obtained by averaging over the counts from the nonattenuated image of the flood source (Figure 5.1).

5.5.1 SPECT Attenuation Correction

SPECT images without attenuation correction show less activity in deep structures than in more superficial regions. This can be approximately corrected by determining the average attenuation that occurs for each voxel by averaging the attenuation across all the lines of detection. This approach requires a map of attenuation coefficients. The simplest method is to assume uniform attenuation across the body. The Chang method uses this assumption in the head and

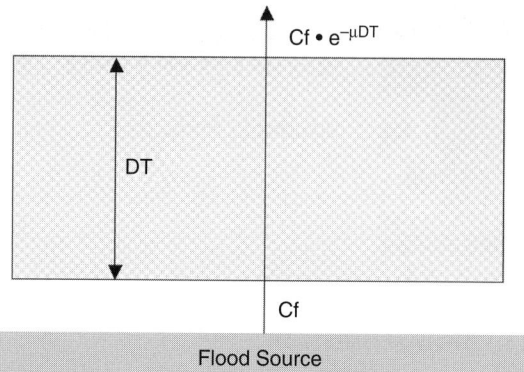

Figure 5.1 Determination of attenuation through an object using a flood source. Cf is the count rate from the flood source without attenuation. $Cf \cdot e^{-\mu DT}$ is the count rate with the attenuation in place. The ratio is $e^{-\mu DT}$ and the square root of the ratio is $e^{-\mu(DT/2)}$. This can be divided into the geometric mean, to yield the attenuation corrected count in units of cpm per pixel. Note that this count represents the attenuation-corrected activity in a column through the patient. It is not proportional to $\mu Ci/ml$; rather it is proportional to the μCi in an area projected through the subject.

is implemented on most SPECT systems. In the head, attenuation is sufficiently uniform that the method works reasonably well. The method requires an outline of the head at each level of interest. This is often constrained to be an ellipse.

The more sophisticated SPECT attenuation correction schemes require a more detailed map of attenuation coefficients. Ideally the map would be obtained from transmission imaging using the same isotope as will be studied. In practice this is difficult to achieve and usually different energies are used for emission and transmission imaging, for example Tc-99m emission and Gd-153 transmission. There are several approximations that are necessarily involved in this approach that result in significant uncertainty.

5.5.2 Positron Emission Tomography Attenuation Correction

A distinct technical advantage of PET imaging over SPECT and planar nuclear medicine approaches is the more accurate attenuation correction. The more accurate attenuation correction arises from the physics of PET imaging that requires detection of two photons. Attenuation is the same at any point along a line of detection and so can be accurately calculated from either a rotating rod source of Ge-68 or with a co-registered CT, after appropriate correction for the different attenuation coefficients of X-rays and 511 keV photons.

5.6 Standardized Uptake Value (SUV)

SUV is overwhelmingly the most commonly used method to assess FDG uptake in PET imaging. It is relatively easy to do, but there are numerous potential problems. The most significant are listed:

1. The PET scanner must be accurately calibrated so that (counts per voxel) per (μCi/ml) is known and entered into the software.
2. The injected dose must be accurately known. This means measuring both the dose syringe prior to injection and any residual activity in tubing and syringe after injection in a dose calibrator.
3. The patients serum glucose level must be measured. Most sites will not image if the serum glucose level is above 200 mg/dl.
4. SUV changes with time. This means imaging should be done at a consistent time. Sixty minutes has become a common time to start imaging, although many sites have changed to imaging at ninety minutes.
5. Infiltrated doses are a major problem. There is no easy correction because of uncertainly regarding the time course of the injection.

Occasionally FDG SUV values seem to be wrong for no discernable cause. The patient weight, administered dose, and times should all be checked. An internal test for reasonableness of SUV values is to check the average SUV in the liver. SUV_{avg} for liver should be in the range of 1.6–2.5.

In PET imaging SUV_{max} is often used as a measure of activity in objects showing increased uptake. The rationale is that it is likely to more closely reflect the true activity in the tissue than average activity in a larger region and that the level of peak activity is the best measure of the metabolic activity of the tissue. One concern regarding SUVmax is that, because of noise, the values may occasionally be spuriously high. One suggestion for dealing with this problem is to use SUVpeak, which is the highest average count in a one cm diameter sphere within a lesion. Many of the newer PET imaging programs have the ability to measure SUVpeak, although the exact implementation may vary among manufacturers.

5.7 Simplified Kinetic Analysis

A method that is slightly more complex than SUV is the simplified kinetic analysis (SKA) method. This approach is based on a widely used expression for tissue uptake of activity, that is the microsphere formula. This approach is superior to the SUV approach since it relates tissue uptake to the availability of tracer to the tissue via the bloodstream. The SUV approach implicitly assumes the injected activity is uniformly available in all patients in the same way, which is probably not true. The formula used is:

$$MR_{SKA} = \frac{Tissue\ activity\ at\ time\ \ t}{Integral\ of\ blood\ activity\ until\ time\ \ t} = \frac{A(t)}{\int_0^t B(t)dt}$$

This requires arterial blood sampling from the time of injection until completion of the PET image. The simplification, introduced by Hunter et al., was to use an average blood TAC for calculating the integral instead of a specific blood TAC for each individual subject. The average blood TAC is scaled to intersect the value obtained from a venous blood sample taken at some time between 45 and 60 minutes after injection. It is assumed that venous activity is essentially equal to arterial activity at late times (Figure 5.2).

5.8 Patlak Graphical Analysis

The graphical approach for the determination of the uptake rates of FDG was developed by Patlak et al. and others to analyze FDG uptake without resorting to compartmental models and parameter optimization. The method requires an arterial plasma time-activity curve and multiple tissue concentrations. The minimal data required is at least one blood sample used to scale an average plasma time-activity curve and PET images at a minimum of two times. The major assumption of this approach is that tracer uptake within tissue is unidirectional without backflux. FDG comes quite close to fitting this assumption in tumors where there is little phosphatase activity but the assumption is less valid in other tissues, such as normal liver where FDG-6-PO$_4$ is rapidly de-phosphorylated back to FDG.

If uptake is unidirectional then the following equation should describe uptake as a function of time:

$$A(t) = V_D \cdot C_B(t) + K \cdot \int_0^t C_B(\tau)d\tau$$

After dividing through by $C_B(t)$:

$$\frac{A(t)}{C_B(t)} = V_D + K \cdot \frac{\int_0^t C_B(\tau)d\tau}{C_B(t)}$$

or, more simply: $A_{norm}(t) = V_D + K\ \theta$

25

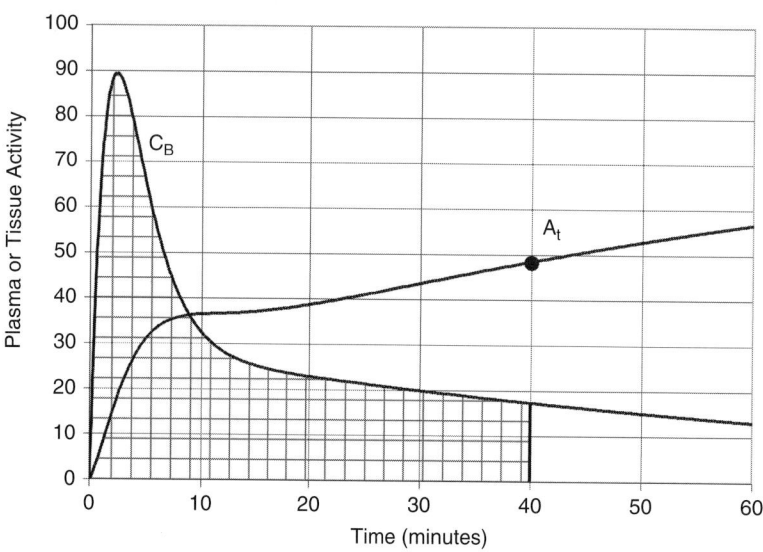

Figure 5.2 Simplified kinetic analysis (simulated data). Tissue uptake (A_t) is normalized by dividing by the area under the blood time-activity (C_B) curve, that is by the hatched area.

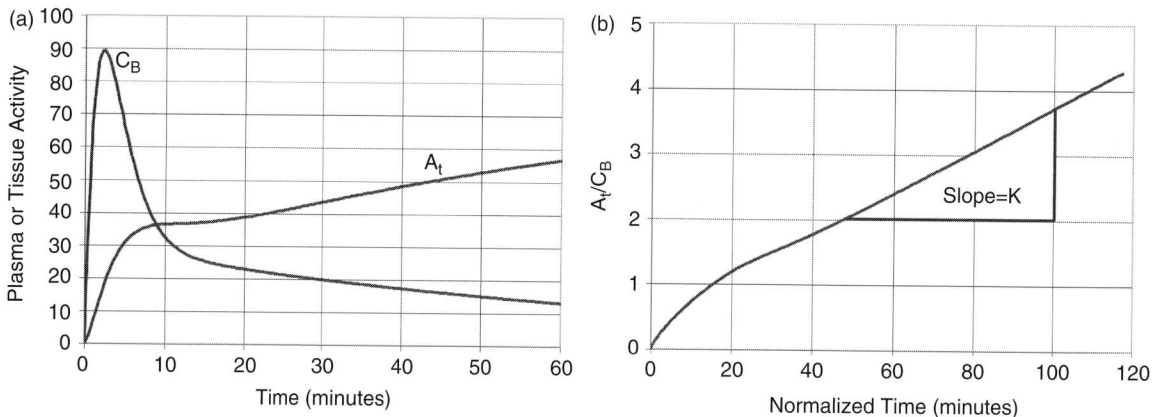

Figure 5.3 Patlak graphical analysis (simulated data). The blood and tissue time-activity curves (A: on the left) are transformed to the ratio of tissue to blood activity (A_t / C_B) and to normalized time, θ. The tissue:blood ratio is plotted against normalized time (B: on the right). After equilibration, the slope of the plot, K, is the metabolic rate of FDG.

where normalized tissue activity, $A_{norm}(t)$, is tissue activity divided by blood activity and θ is normalized time, that is

$$\theta = \frac{\int_0^t C_B(\tau)d\tau}{C_B(t)}$$

In the Patlak plot, $A_{norm}(t)$ is plotted (vertically) versus normalized time (θ) (horizontally). The slope after equilibration is K and the intercept is V_D. This method can be used with the scaled population blood TAC similar to the way it was used for simplified kinetic analysis (Figure 5.3). FDG metabolic rate is the product of K times plasma glucose level.

Further Reading

Chang LT. A method of attenuation correction in radionuclide computed tomography. *IEEE Trans Nucl Sci.* 25:638–43.

Hamberg LM, Hunter GJ, Alpert NM, Choi NC, Babich JW, Fischman AJ. The dose uptake ratio as an index of glucose metabolism: useful parameter or oversimplification? *J Nucl Med.* 1994 Aug;35(8):1308–12.

Keyes JW Jr. SUV: standard uptake or silly useless value? *J Nucl Med.* 1995 Oct;36(10):1836–9.

Wahl RL, Jacene H, Kasamon Y, Lodge MA. From RECIST to PERCIST: Evolving Considerations for PET response criteria in solid tumors. *J Nucl Med.* 2009 May;50 Suppl 1:122S–50S.

Hunter GJ, Hamberg LM, Alpert NM, Choi NC, Fischman AJ. Simplified measurement of deoxyglucose utilization rate. *J Nucl Med.* 1996 Jun;37(6):950–5.

Graham MM, Peterson LM, Hayward RM. Comparison of simplified quantitative analyses of FDG uptake. *Nucl Med Biol.* 2000 Oct;27(7):647–55.

Patlak CS, Blasberg RG, and Fenstermacher JD. Graphical evaluation of blood-to-brain transfer constants from multiple-time uptake data. *J Cereb Blood Flow Metab.* 1983. 3:1–7.

Gjedde, A. Calculation of cerebral glucose phosphorylation from brain uptake of glucose analogs in vivo: a re-examination. *Brain Res Rev.* 1982. 4:237–74.

Perfusion

Michael Graham

Perfusion is usually defined as the capillary blood flow to tissue, and is expressed in milliliter per gram per minute. A typical value for myocardial perfusion at rest is 0.5–1.0 ml/g/min and for brain is 0.4–0.6 ml/g/min. Perfusion may be different from the blood flow to a tissue if there is significant arteriovenous shunting.

6.1 Microspheres

The gold standard for perfusion measurements in experimental animals is the microsphere method. This approach is not used in human studies. Microspheres are small spheres, 15–25 microns in diameter, labeled with either radioactive or fluorescent tracers. Radioactive microspheres are currently available in the United States from only one company, Perkin-Elmer. An alternative to microspheres is Tc-99m macroaggregated albumin, which is used clinically for perfusion lung scans. Tissue and blood activity is determined by counting with a scintillation well counter. Fluorescent microspheres are available from several manufacturers. Tissue and blood activity is determined using a fluorescent spectrophotometer, although other methods have also been used.

Ideally a catheter is positioned in the left atrium to ensure optimal mixing, and the microspheres are infused at a constant rate for a short period, perhaps one minute. Beginning immediately before the infusion, a syringe pump is started, which withdraws arterial blood at a constant rate during the microsphere infusion, and is stopped 30–60 seconds after the end of the infusion. The syringe pump acts as an "artificial organ" with known blood flow. The activity in the syringe is determined and then acts as a standard to compare to tissue samples.

Example: The syringe pump withdraws blood at 1 ml/min and the activity in the syringe at the end of the experiment is determined to be 1,000 counts per minute (CPM). If a sample of muscle weighs 2 g and

has 100 CPM, then the entire piece has blood flow of 0.1 ml/min and the perfusion is 0.05 ml/g/min.

A different approach for using microspheres is to take blood samples rapidly during the infusion. Then blood flow to an organ is calculated by dividing the tissue activity by the integral area under the blood time activity curve. The flow to tissue sample J with tissue activity concentration C_J is:

$$Flow_J = \frac{C_J(T)}{\int_0^T C_B(t)dt}$$

where C_B is the concentration of activity in arterial blood.

6.2 Myocardial Perfusion

Microspheres have been used in animal studies of myocardial perfusion, although studies in humans have used less invasive methods. Several radio-labeled tracers are used in clinical studies, as well as in research settings. All of the tracers used are taken up rapidly and most can be imaged several minutes later, after most activity has cleared from the blood. An ideal tracer would have complete uptake as it moves through the capillary bed. All of the available tracers are less than ideal and significant correction is necessary to use them to quantitate myocardial blood flow. The newest of the tracers, depicted in Figure 6.1, is F-18 flurpiridaz, which is still in clinical trial, but is likely to be approved for human use in the near future.

6.3 Cerebral Perfusion with Retained Agents

Currently Tc-99m hexamethylpropyleneamine oxime (HMPAO), also called exametazime, and Tc-99m ethyl cysteinate dimer (ECD) are the only approved

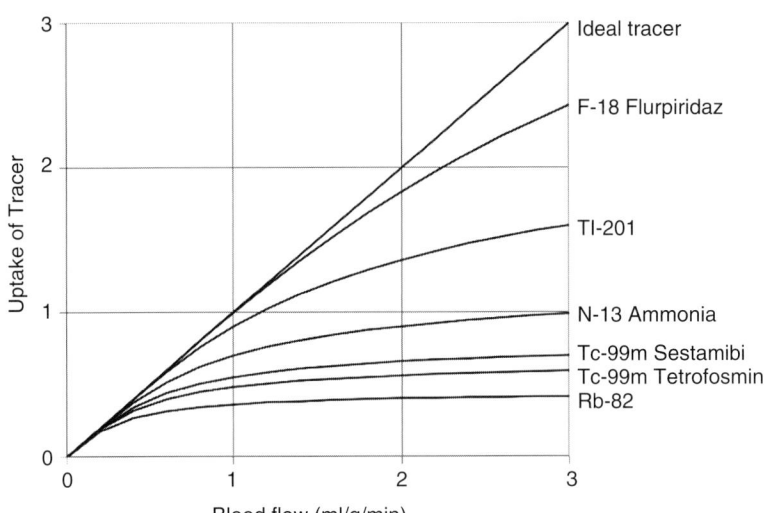

Figure 6.1 Approximate myocardial uptake curves for common myocardial perfusion agents.

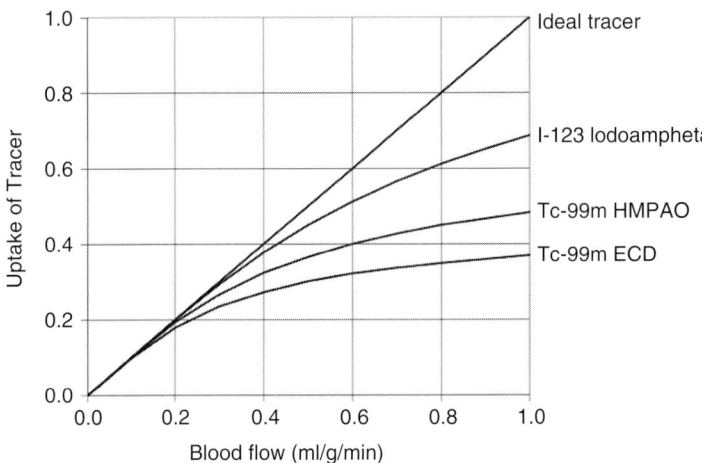

Figure 6.2 Approximate brain uptake curves for common cerebral perfusion agents

agents for cerebral perfusion in the US. I-123 iodo-amphetamine (IMP) was available in the past in the United States and continues to be used in other countries, particularly in Japan (Figure 6.2).

Both agents are lipophilic and are rapidly taken up into the brain proportional to blood flow. Clinical imaging of these agents is done with single photon emission computed tomography (SPECT). The images are useful for evaluation of relative blood flow, but are not generally quantitated. If accurate tissue quantitation is available, by tissue sampling or with attenuation-corrected SPECT, perfusion can be calculated with the microsphere formula, with correction for incomplete extraction.

6.4 Cerebral Perfusion with Diffusible Agents

There are several agents that have much higher extraction fractions than the retained agents discussed previously. Three of the most commonly used highly diffusible agents are O-15 water, X-133 Xenon, and I-123 iodoantipyrine. There are several major methods used to measure blood flow with these agents. Five of the commonly used approaches are:

- Indicator fractionation.
  - This approach is commonly used with iodoantipyine in mice or rats. The agent is injected intravenously as a very rapid bolus,

arterial blood is constantly withdrawn, as in a microsphere experiment. Typically at about ten seconds after the bolus injection the animal is decapitated and blood withdrawal is stopped, before any activity has left the brain. Activity in the brain is determined and blood flow is calculated with the microsphere formula. Regional blood flow can be determined using quantitative autoradiography.

- Tissue equilibration.
  - This approach is also used in small animals. The agent is injected intravenously over 30–60 seconds, using a steadily increasing infusion rate. Rapid arterial blood sampling is done and the animal is decapitated at the end of the study. Activity in the brain is determined and blood flow can be calculated using an established model for the behavior of diffusible agents. Regional blood flow can be determined using quantitative autoradiography.
- Equilibration with short-lived tracers.
  - A short-lived diffusible tracer (e.g. O-15 water, or O-15 carbon dioxide, which is converted in the lungs to water via carbonic anhydrase) is infused at a constant rate. After 4–5 half-lives, equilibration is achieved, where the tracer is decaying as fast as it is being delivered. It is then possible to calculate absolute blood flow from a PET image of the brain. These studies have been used in animals and humans.
- Compartmental modeling approach.
  - O-15 water or another detectable, freely diffusible agent is injected intravenously, followed by arterial blood sampling and imaging. Using a one-compartment model, and accounting for tracer decay, it is possible to accurately estimate regional cerebral blood flow. This method is the most widely used approach for quantitation of cerebral blood flow in humans.
- Washout of diffusible agents.
  - Following intra-arterial administration of a diffusible agent, activity in the tissue will decrease in an exponential fashion. The time constant (min^{-1}), after appropriate correction for partition coefficient and tissue density, is the tissue perfusion ($ml\ g^{-1}\ min^{-1}$).

This approach also works with inhaled Xe-133, since there is minimal recirculation. Most activity in venous blood is exhaled. A variation on this approach is to use direct injection of Xe-133 dissolved in saline into a tissue (e.g. muscle or tumor) and then to measure the washout time constant. These studies have been used in animals and humans.

6.5 Cerebral Blood Flow with MRI

The most widely used technique with MRI uses the blood oxygen level dependent (BOLD) signal. This is an indirect measure of blood flow, in that the signal depends on the change in oxygen level, which is assumed to decrease shortly after neuronal activation, which elicits an increase in blood flow. The relationship between MRI signal and blood flow is nonlinear and is used qualitatively to identify regions of increased blood flow in response to a stimulus.

Another MRI method is arterial spin labeling (ASL). The protons in arterial blood, that is water, are spin labeled in the arteries in the neck. The subsequent changes in signal in the cerebral cortex can be used to provide a measure of cerebral blood flow. The method is similar to the O-15 water approach, but the instrumentation and corrections are quite different. An advantage of this technique is that it is quantitative, although it tends to overestimate cerebral blood flow.

6.6 Cerebral Blood Flow with CT

Measurement of regional blood flow with CT is used particularly in the evaluation of acute stroke. Dynamic CT images are acquired immediately following IV bolus injection of contrast. Time-density curves are determined for arteries, veins, and brain parenchyma. Calculation of cerebral blood flow is based on the central volume principle, which assumes the tracer is distributed in a constant volume, in this case the vascular volume of the brain. The relationship is then CBF = CBV/ MTT. CBF is cerebral blood flow (ml/g/min). CBV is cerebral blood volume (Ml/g). MTT is mean transit time (min), which is derived from a deconvolution of the tissue time-density curve with the arterial time density curve. Typical MTT for normal brain is about six seconds. The data is usually displayed as a parametric, color-coded images of CBF, CBV, or MTT.

Further Reading

Anderson RE. Cerebral blood flow xenon-133. *Neurosurg Clin N Am*. 1996;7(4):703–8.

Frackowiak RSJ, Lenzi G-L, Jones T, Heather JD. Quantitative measurement of regional cerebral blood flow and oxygen metabolism in man using O-15 and positron emission tomography: Theory, procedure, and normal values. *J Comput Assist Tomogr*. 1980 4:727–36.

Golay X, Hendrikse J, Lim TC. Perfusion imaging using arterial spin labeling. *Top Magn Reson Imaging*. 2004; 15(1):10–27.

Harris JJ, Reynell C, Attwell D. The physiology of developmental changes in BOLD functional imaging signals. *Dev Cogn Neurosci*. 2011; 1(3):199–216.

Huang SC, Carson RE, Hoffman EJ, Carson J, MacDonald N, Barrio JR, Phelps ME. Quantitative measurement of local cerebral blood flow in humans by positron computed tomography and 15O-water. *J Cereb Blood Flow Metab*. 1983;3(2):141–53.

Nabavi DG, Cenic A, Craen RA, Gelb AW, Bennett JD, Kozak R, Lee TY. CT assessment of cerebral perfusion: experimental validation and initial clinical experience. *Radiology*. 1999; 213(1):141–9.

Patlak CS, Blasberg RG, Fenstermacher JD. An evaluation of errors in the determination of blood flow by the indicator fractionation and tissue equilibration (Kety) methods. *J Cereb Blood Flow Metab*. 1984 Mar;4(1):47–60.

Prinzen FW, Bassingthwaighte JB. Blood flow distributions by microsphere deposition methods. *Cardiovasc Res*. 2000 Jan 1;45(1):13–21.

Chapter

7

Metabolism

Hossein Jadvar

7.1 Glucose

Glucose is a major source of energy in many organisms. Processing of glucose may involve aerobic or anaerobic respiration with the purpose of producing energy in the form of adenosine-5'-triphosphate (ATP), a recycled molecular currency for cellular transfer of energy. The first step in both aeorobic and anaeroobic glucose metabolism is phosphorylation by hexokinase forming glucose-6-phosphate. In humans, the two major routes for further processing of the glucose-6-phosphate are eventual formation and storage of glycogen in the liver as stored energy or propagation toward the citric acid cycle with eventual production of CO_2 and water. In aerobic respiration a molecule of glucose produces a net of 32 ATP molecules while anaerobic glucose metabolism generates a net of only 2 ATP molecules.

Glucose has played a key role in molecular imaging with positron emission tomography (PET) since the time when an analog of glucose was radiolabeled with the positron emitter, fluorine-18 that substituted for the 2' position in the glucose molecule. This glucose analog, 2-deoxy-2-(^{18}F)fluoro-D-glucose, abbreviated as FDG, enabled the imaging evaluation of glucose metabolism in health and disease. FDG PET has now unequivocally revolutionized clinical practice for a number of applications, most notably in cancer.

It has long been known that most tumors are hypermetabolic, with increased glucose metabolism (Warburg effect). The underlying mechanism and reason for elevated glucose metabolism in cancers is multifactorial and may relate to tumor-related factors (e.g. type and histologic differentiation), biochemical and molecular alterations (e.g. hypoxia), and nontumor-related components (e.g. inflammation). It has been proposed that the relationship between tumor growth and glucose metabolism may be explained in terms of adaptation to hypoxia through upregulation of glucose transporters (GLUTs) and increased enzymatic activity of hexokinase, as one of the "hallmarks of cancer."

Glucose is transported across the cell via a family of fourteen facilitative GLUTs that are cell-specific and affected by hormonal and environmental factors. A list of these facilitative GLUTs can be found at www.genenames.org/cgi-bin/hgnc_search.pl (N.B. the currently approved gene symbol is SLC2Ax). The enhanced tumor glucose metabolism is associated with overexpression of primarily hypoxia-responsive GLUT1 or GLUT3 proteins. Increased hexokinase type II (of the four types in mammalian tissue) enzymatic level and activity has also been implicated in many cancers. FDG is phosphorylated to FDG-6-phosphate, but contrary to glucose-6-phosphate, it cannot be metabolized further in the glycolytic metabolic pathway and becomes trapped in the cell. The low activity of the reverse enzyme, glucose-6-phophatase, in most tumor cells also contributes to the tumor cell accumulation of FDG-6-phosphate that is then imaged with PET.

Normal biodistribution of FDG shows high uptake in the brain grey matter, lactating breast, thymus and growth plates in children, and in the excreted urine spaces (e.g. renal pelvis, along ureters, urinary bladder), variable uptake in the heart and bowel, mild uptake in the normal liver, and relatively lower uptake than liver in the other tissues (Figure 7.1).

The major clinical applications of FDG PET(/CT) are in neurology (e.g. Alzheimer dementia, seizure focus localization), cardiology (e.g. myocardial viability), and oncology. In fact, FDG PET(/CT) has revolutionized the imaging evaluation of patients with cancer and is now routinely used in the clinic for a variety of indications in a number of common cancers (e.g. lung, breast, colon, head and neck, esophagus, lymphoma, etc.). The main indications have included diagnosis, staging, restaging, evaluating treatment response, and assessing prognosis. However, it should

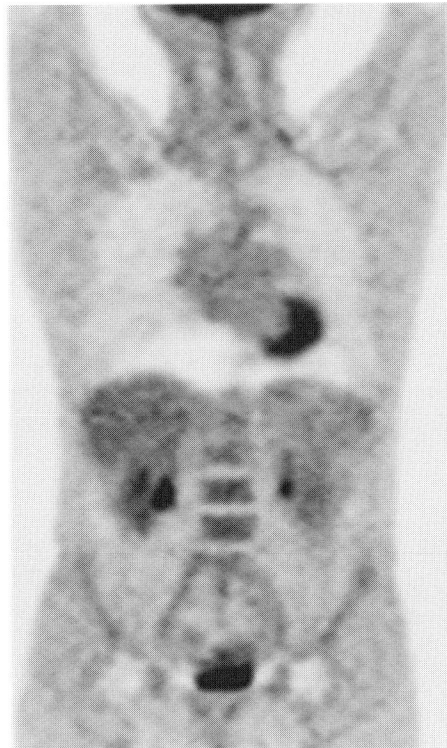

Figure 7.1 Normal biodistribution FDG (Kostakoglu L et al. *Radiographics* 2004).

be noted that FDG is not cancer-specific and benign conditions such as inflammation and infection can accumulate FDG. Although this may initially seem as a limitation in the imaging evaluation of patients with suspected or known cancer, in those patients without cancer, FDG PET(/CT) may in fact be useful in assessing the extent of inflammatory disease and/or response to relevant treatments.

7.2 Acetate

Acetate is a simple metabolite that is preferentially transported across the cellular membrane through the monocarboxylate transporter. The two major sources of acetate consumption are the citric acid cycle and the metabolic pathways related to the production of phospholipids in cellular membranes facilitated by the fatty acid synthase (FAS) reaction that is upregulated in malignancy.

Acetate may be radiolabeled with carbon-11 (^{11}C) or fluorine-18 (^{18}F). However, the majority of PET studies have been performed with the ^{11}C label. Normal biodistribution of ^{11}C-acetate displays high accumulation in the pancreas, variable uptake in the liver and bowel, and some renal uptake with little urinary excretion (Figure 7.2).

Similar to FDG, ^{11}C-actete is not cancer-specific and benign conditions (e.g. meningioma, thymoma, atherosclerosis) can accumulate the tracer. The major cancers that have been studied with ^{11}C-acetate PET(/CT) have included glioma, bronchoalveolar carcinoma, hepatocellular carcinoma, renal cell carcinoma, and prostate cancer, often providing complementary information to FDG PET(/CT).

7.3 Choline

Choline enters the cell through choline transporters and is the precursor for the biosynthesis of phospholipids which are major components of the cellular membrane. The biological basis for the accumulation of radiolabeled choline in tumors is in part due to malignancy-induced overexpression of choline kinase in support of increased demand for cellular membrane synthesis. Choline kinase catalyzes the phosphorylation of choline to form phosphorylcholine followed by generation of phosphatidylcholine in the tumor cell membrane.

Initial studies with choline were performed with ^{11}C as the radiolabel. Normal biodistribution of ^{11}C-choline demonstrates relatively high accumulation in the pancreas, liver, kidneys, salivary glands, and variable uptake in the bowel and little urinary excretion. More recently, an ^{18}F-labeled formulation of choline has also become available and in general may be preferred over the ^{11}C label in view of the longer half life of ^{18}F in comparison to [11]C (Figure 7.3). Normal biodistribution of ^{18}F-fluorocholine shows relatively high uptake in the pancreas, liver, spleen, kidneys, variable uptake in the bowel and excretion into urine (Figure 7.4).

Again similar to FDG and ^{11}C-acetate, radiolabeled choline is not cancer-specific. Benign conditions such as thymoma, paraganglioma, meningioma, and atherosclerosis can accumulate the tracer. The major cancers that have been studied with choline include brain, thyroid, lung, esophagus, hepatocellular carcinoma, bladder, and prostate. However, of all these cancers, prostate cancer has received intense attention over the past several years spearheaded by the European and Japanese investigators. Particularly, ^{18}F-fluorocholine PET(/CT) may soon be adopted for imaging evaluation of men with biochemical relapse of prostate cancer and negative standard of care imaging studies.

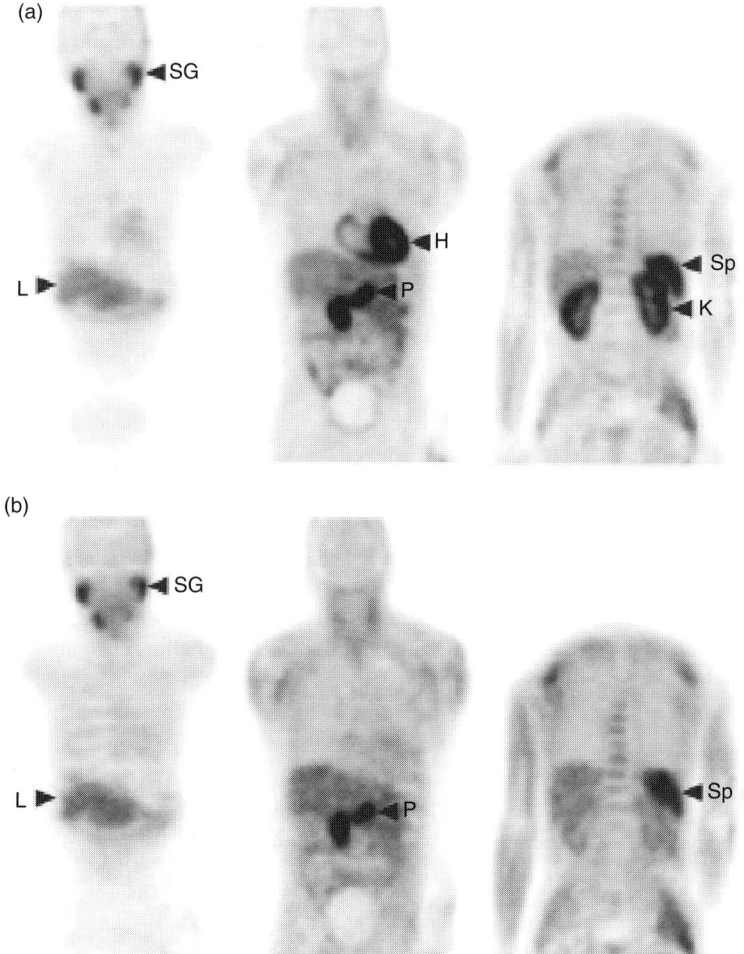

Figure 7.2 Normal biodistribution of 11C-acetate (Czernin J et al. *PET Clin* 2009).

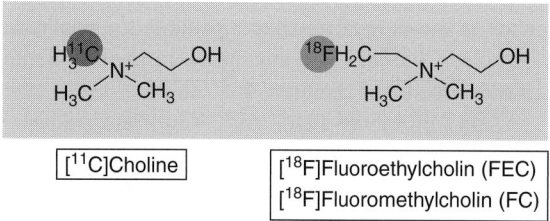

[11C]Choline

[18F]Fluoroethylcholin (FEC)
[18F]Fluoromethylcholin (FC)

Figure 7.3 The chemical structures of ^{11}C-choline and ^{18}F-fluorocholine (Courtesy of Dr. Bernd J. Krause, University of Rostock, Germany).

Further Reading

Basu S, Alavi A. Revolutionary impact of PET and PET-CT on the day-to-day practice of medicine and its great potential for improving future health care. *Nucl Med Rev Cent East Eur* 2009; 12:1–13.

DeGrado TR, Coleman RE, Wang S, Baldwin SW, Orr MD, Robertson CN, et al. Synthesis and evaluation of 18F-labeled choline as an oncologic tracer for positron emission tomography: initial findings in prostate cancer. *Cancer Res* 2001; 61(1):110–17.

Gillies RJ, Robey I, Gatenby RA. Causes and consequences of increased glucose metabolism of cancers. *J Nucl Med* 2008; 49(6 suppl):24S–42S.

Hanahan D, Weinberg RA. The hallmarks of cancer: the next generation. *Cell* 2011; 144:646–74.

Jadvar H, Alavi A, Gambhir SS. 18F-FDG uptake in lung, breast, and colon cancers: molecular biology correlates and disease characterization. *J Nucl Med* 2009; 50:1820–27.

Janardhan S, Srivani P, Sastry GN. Choline kinase: an important target for cancer. *Curr Med Chem* 2006; 13:1169–86.

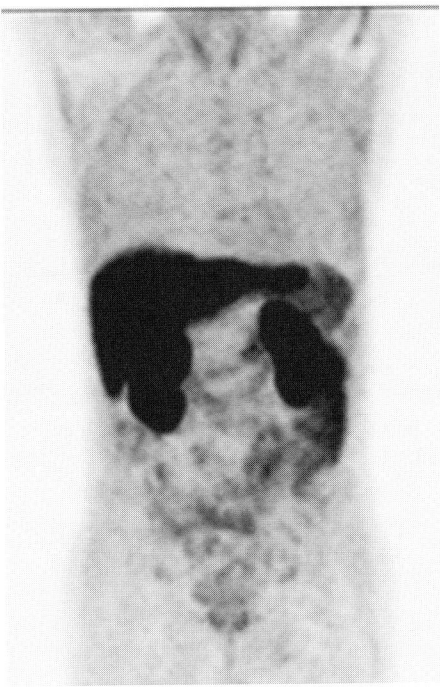

Figure 7.4 Normal biodistribution of ^{11}C-choline (Yanagawa T et al. *J Comput Assist Tomogr* 2003).

Macheda ML, Rogers S, Bets JD. Molecular and cellular regulation of glucose transport (GLUT) proteins in cancer. *J Cell Physiol* 2005; 202:654–62.

Picchio M, Briganti A, Fanti S, Fanti S, Heidenreich A, Krause BJ, et al. The role of choline positron emission tomography/computed tomography in the management of patients with prostate-specific antigen progression after radical treatment of prostate cancer. *Eur Urol* 2011; 59:51–60.

Ponde DE, Dence CS, Oyama N, Kim J, Tai YC, Laforest R, et al. 18F-fluoroacetate: a potential acetate analog for prostate tumors imaging – in vivo evaluation of 18F-fluoroacetate versus 11C-acetate. *J Nucl Med* 2007; 48:420–8.

Reischl G, Bieg C, Schmiedl O, Solbach C, Machulla HJ. Highly efficient automated synthesis of [(11)C]choline for multi dose utilization. *Appl Radiat Isot* 2004; 60:835–8.

Seltzer MA, Jahan SA, Sparks R, Stout DB, Satyamurthy N, Dahlborn, et al. Radiation dose estimates in humans for (11)C-acetate whole-body PET. *J Nucl Med* 2004; 45(7):1233–6.

Smith TA. Mammalian hexokinases and their abnormal expression in cancer. *Br J Biomed Sci* 2000; 57:170–8.

Vander Heiden MG, Cantley LC, Thompson CB. Understanding the Warburg effect: the metabolic requirements of cell proliferation. *Science* 324: 1029–33.

Yoshimoto M, Waki A, Yonekura Y, Sadato N, Murata T, Omata N, et al. Characterization of acetate metabolism in tumor cells in relation to cell proliferation: acetate metabolism in tumor cells. *Nucl Med Biol* 2001; 28:117–22.

Cellular Proliferation

Hossein Jadvar

Controlled proliferation is an important physiologic cellular function. However, uncontrolled cellular proliferation is one of the major hallmarks of cancer. Imaging cellular proliferation may provide valuable diagnostic information about the rate of tumor growth and an opportunity for objective assessment of early response to treatment. Positron emission tomography (PET) in conjunction with radiotracers that track the thymidine salvage pathway of DNA synthesis has been studied extensively for imaging cellular proliferation in cancer. Initially, [^{11}C-methyl]thymidine ([^{11}C-methl]TdR) was synthesized for this purpose but the radiotracer had the major limitation of rapid catabolism. Further research resulted in the development of new radiolabeled analogs that were resistant to catabolism. Those radiotracers labeled with ^{18}F are of particular interest since the longer isotope half-life (110 min) facilitates regional distribution of the tracer without the need for an on-site cyclotron. In this chapter, we briefly describe the experience with two of these radiotracers, [^{18}F]-3'-deoxy-3'-fluorothymidine (^{18}F-FLT) and [^{18}F]-2'-fluoro-5-methyl-1-beta-D-arabinofuranosyluracil (^{18}F-FMAU) (Figure 8.1).

8.1 [^{18}F]-FLT

^{18}F-FLT is the most studied cellular proliferation PET tracer. The radiotracer is phosphorylated by thymidine kinase 1 (TK1), retained in proliferating cells without DNA incorporation, and can be described by a three-compartment model. Normal biodistribution of ^{18}F-FLT demonstrates relatively high uptake in the liver and the bone marrow with urinary bladder receiving the highest dose through renal excretion. Typically ^{18}F-FLT demonstrates lower uptake than ^{18}F-FDG in tumors, although in some anatomic regions, such as the brain, the target-to-background uptake ratio is higher with ^{18}F-FLT than with FDG (given the high physiologic FDG uptake in the brain gray matter). Tehrani and Shields recently summarized the literature on the major clinical investigations with ^{18}F-FLT. These authors caution that not all tumors with high proliferation may show high ^{18}F-FLT uptake due to a variety of factors including the type of cancer and treatment, and biologic processes such as balance between de novo and salvage pathways of DNA synthesis, and balance between increased proliferation rate and decreased apoptosis.

The low ^{18}F-FLT uptake in the normal brain is an advantage that has been investigated for the grading of brain tumors, differentiation of radiation necrosis from residual or recurrent tumor, assessment of treatment response, and in prognostication. However, one must note that ^{18}F-FLT does not cross the blood-brain barrier and hence tumor uptake of ^{18}F-FLT may represent a combination of tumor tracer localization from the barrier breakdown and the tracer accumulation in tumor cells reflecting cellular proliferation.

In head and neck cancer, ^{18}F-FLT has been found to have a competitive advantage over FDG for the differentiation of neoplastic and inflammatory nodal involvement. This is based on the lower ^{18}F-FLT uptake in inflammatory processes, providing higher specificity than FDG in this setting. ^{18}F-FLT has therefore been considered more useful than FDG for early follow-up after radiation treatment in head and neck cancer.

Lung cancer and lymphoma have been studied relatively extensively with ^{18}F-FLT. In both cancers, the level of tracer accumulation in tumor is generally correlated with the cellular proliferation index, Ki-67. In comparison to FDG, ^{18}F-FLT demonstrates lower sensitivity, higher specificity, and higher positive predictive value. Early decline in tumor uptake of ^{18}F-FLT in response to treatment may also be predictive of longer progression-free survival.

8.2 ^{18}F-FMAU

Unlabeled FMAU was originally of clinical interest as an anticancer and an antiviral drug when used in

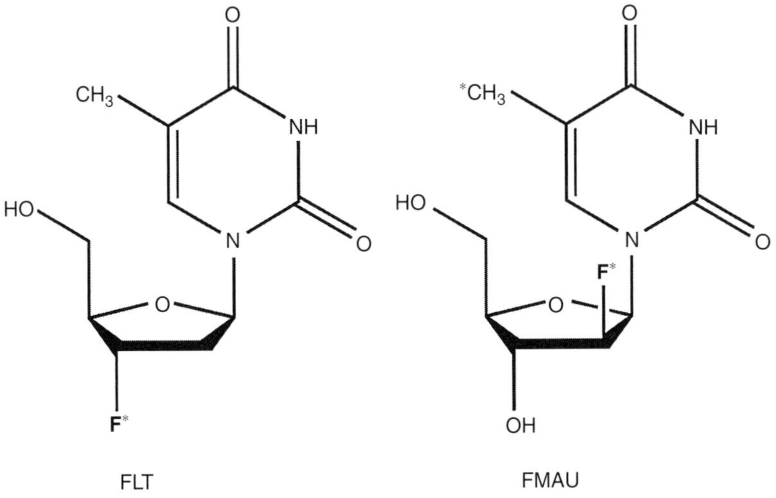

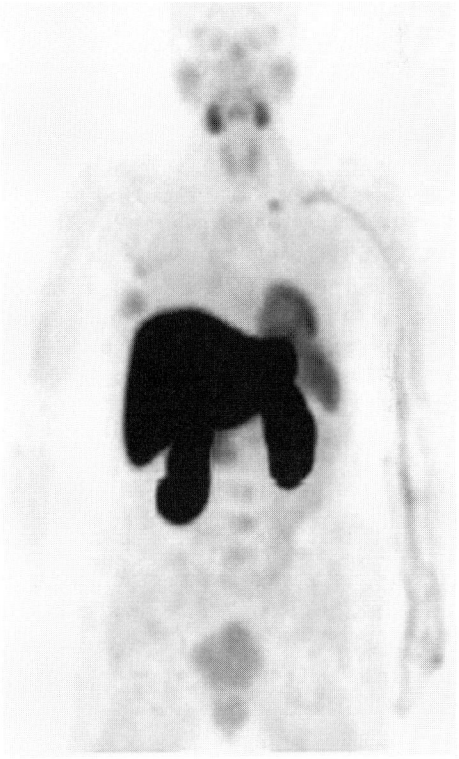

Figure 8.1 Chemical structures of ^{18}F-FLT and ^{18}F-FMAU (adapted from Ref. 6 and used with permission). *F denotes the position of [18]F.

FLT   FMAU

pharmacological doses. It is a thymidine analog that is phosphorylated by both cytosol TK1 and mitochondrial TK2 and incorporated into the DNA (an advantage over ^{18}F-FLT which does not incorporate into DNA at all), reflecting the same DNA synthetic pathway as thymidine in proportion to the rate of proliferation. Indeed, it has been shown that at least about 10 per cent of ^{18}F-FMAU is incorporated into the DNA by ten minutes after tracer administration; highly proliferative tumors are also under 'cellular stress' reflected in increased mitochondrial TK2 activity and hence increased ^{18}F-FMAU trapping. TK2 has an important role in replication and maintenance of mitochondrial DNA. Pharmacokinetic studies have shown that ^{14}C-FMAU behaves very similar to the pyrimidine nucleoside, thymidine, with respect to cellular uptake velocity, saturability of cellular incorporation, and intracellular metabolite pools and is reflective of tumor cell division. The adequacy of three-compartment model has also been shown for FMAU. Normal biodistribution of ^{18}F-FMAU demonstrates relatively high tracer uptake in the liver and the renal cortex, moderate uptake in the salivary glands, heart, and spleen and relatively low uptake in the bone marrow (Figure 8.2). ^{18}F-FMAU has not been studied extensively in the clinical arena, although it has been evaluated in a few preclinical and pilot clinical investigations.

Further Reading

1. Hanahan D, Weinberg RA. Hallmarks of cancer: the next generation. *Cell* 2011; 144:646–74.

Figure 8.2 Normal biodistribution of ^{18}F-FMAU in human (adapted from Ref. 6 and used with permission).

2. Mankoff DA, Shields AF, Krohn KA. PET imaging of cellular proliferation. *Radiol Clin North Am* 2005; 43:153–67.

3. Couturier O, Leost F, Campone M, Cartlier T, Chatal JF, Hustinx R. Is 3'-deoxy-3'-[18F]fluorothymidine

([18F]-FLT) the next tracer for routine clinical PET after [18F]-FDG? *Bull Cancer* 2005; 92:789–98.

4. Nimmagadda S, Shields AF. The role of DNA synthesis imaging in cancer in the era of targeted therapeutics. *Cancer Metastasis Rev* 2008; 27:575–87.

5. Krohn KA, Mankoff DA, Eary JF. Imaging cellular proliferation as measure of response to therapy. *J Clin Pharmacol* 2011; Suppl:96S–103S.

6. Bading JR, Shields AF. Imaging of cell proliferation: status and prospects. *J Nucl Med* 2008; 49 Suppl 2:64S–80S.

7. Christman D, Crawford EJ, Friedkin M, Wolf AP. Detection of DNA synthesis in intact organisms with positron-emitting (methyl-11C)thymidine. *Proc Natl Acad Sci USA* 1972; 69:988–92.

8. Shields AF, Mankoff DA, Graham MM, Zheng M, Lozawa SM, Link JM et al. Analysis of 2-carbon-11-thymidine blood metabolites in PET imaging. *J Nucl Med* 1996; 37:290–6.

9. Shields AF, Mankoff DA, Link JM, Graham MM, Eary JF, Kozawa SM et al. [11C]Thymidine and FDG to measure therapy response. *J Nucl Med* 1998; 39:1757–62.

10. Mankoff D, Shields AF, Link JM, Graham MM, Muzi M, Pterson LM et al. Kinetic analysis of 2-[11C] thymidine PET imaging studies: validation studies. *J Nucl Med* 1999; 40:614–24.

11. Mankoff D, Shield AF, Graham MM, Link JM, Eary JF, Krohn KA. Kinetic analysis of 2-[carbon- 11] thymidine PET imaging studies: compartmental model and mathematical analysis. *J Nucl Med* 1998; 39:1043–55.

12. Shields AF, Grierson JR, Muzik O, Stayanoff JC, Lawhorn-Crews JM, Obradovich JE et al. Kinetics of 3'-deoxy-3'-[F- 18]fluorothymidine uptake and retention in dogs. *Mol Imaging Biol* 2002 4:83–9.

13. Shields AF, Briston DA, Chandupatla S, Douglas KA, Lawhorn-Crews J, Collins JM et al. A simplified analysis of [18F]3'- deoxy-3'-fluorthymidine

metabolism and retention. *Eur J Nucl Med Mol Imaging* 2005; 32:1269–75.

14. Shields AF, Grierson J, Dohmen B, Machulla HJ, Stananoff JC, Lawhorn-Crews JM et al. Imaging proliferation in vivo with [F- 18]FLT and positron emission tomography. *Nat Med* 1998; 4:1334–6.

15. Grierson JR, Shields AF. Radiosynthesis of 3'-deoxy-3'-[(18F]fluorothymidine: [(18F)F]FLT for imaging of cellular proliferation in vivo. *Nucl Med Biol* 2000.

16. Vesselle H, Grierson J, Peterson LM, Muzi M, Mankoff DA, Krohn KA. ^{18}F-fluorothymidine radiation dosimetry in human PET imaging studies. *J Nucl Med* 2003; 44:1482–8.

17. Tehrani OS, Shields AF. PET imaging of proliferation with pyrimdines. *J Nucl Med* 2013; 54:903–12.

18. Saga T, Kawashima H, Araki N et al. Evaluation of primary brain tumors with FLT-PET: usefulness and limitations. *Clin Nucl Med* 2006; 31:774–80.

19. Tehrani OS, Douglas KA, Lawhom-Crews JM et al. Tracking cellular stress with labeled FMAU reflects changes in mitochondrial TK2. *Eur J Nucl Med Mol Imaging* 2008; 35:1480–8.

20. Tehrani OS, Muzik O, Heilbrun LK et al. Tumor imaging using 1-(29-deoxy-29-18FFluoro-b-D-Arabinofuranosyl)Thymine and PET. *J Nucl Med* 2007; 48:1436–41.

21. Sun H, Mangner TJ, Collins JM et al. Imaging DNA synthesis in vivo with 18FFMAU and PET. *J Nucl Med* 2005; 46(2):292–6.

22. Sun H, Sloan A, Mangner TJ, Vaishamayan U, Muzik O, Collins JM et al. Imaging DNA synthesis with [18F]FMAU and positron emission tomography in patients with cancer. *Eur J Nucl Med Mol Imaging* 2005; 32:15–22.

23. Jadvar H, Yap L-P, Park R et al. [18F]-2'-fluoro-5-methyl-1-beta-D-arabinofuranosyluracil (18F-FMAU) in prostate cancer: initial preclinical observations. *Mol Imaging* 2012; 11:426–32.

Hypoxia

Michael Graham

Hypoxia is a significant modifier of malignant tumors, generally increasing their resistance to therapy. It has been known for decades that hypoxic tissue is less radiosensitive than normoxic tissue. The ratio of radiation sensitivities between normoxic and hypoxic tissue, also called the oxygen enhancement ratio (OER), can be as high as 3.0. Radiation oncologists recognize this problem and have adapted their treatment methodology, that is fractionation schedules, to take it into account.

However, hypoxia has multiple other effects beyond increasing the radio-resistance of tumors. In the presence of hypoxia, a number of intracellular pathways are activated, leading to increased levels of HIF-1a, which, in turn, activates a large number of genes, leading to increased levels of enzymes that increase glucose metabolism, apoptosis resistance, angiogenesis, and promote invasion and metastases in tumors. In addition, hypoxia is almost always associated with very low blood flow and results in poor delivery of intravenous chemotherapy drugs to the tumor.

9.1 Direct Measurement of Tissue Oxygen

The polarographic oxygen electrode methodology is generally accepted as the gold standard for measuring tissue oxygen levels. A commercially available system is manufactured by Eppendorf. The electrodes consist of a gold cathode with an insulating glass sheath. The cathode tip is recessed and covered by an oxygen permeable membrane, such as Teflon. The anode is silver-silver chloride. The electrode is in the form of a needle, which is slowly advanced into the tissue automatically. Significant problems with this approach are that it is invasive and can be difficult to implement.

Another, more recent oxygen probe is an optical fiber device that has a ruthenium lumiphor incorporated into a silicone polymer at the tip of the probe. Light pulses through the optical fiber induce fluorescence of the lumiphor, which can be detected. The lifetime of the fluorescent pulses is inversely related to the oxygen level at the tip.

9.2 Magnetic Resonance Spectroscopy (MRS)

An important subset of genes up-regulated by HIF-1a are the genes coding for glycolytic enzymes, such as lactate dehydrogenase and pyruvate dehydrogenase kinase. Their increased activity increases tumor glycolysis, along with increased production of lactate. The concentration of lactate can be estimated, using proton MRS, and this has been used to identify areas of hypoxia within tumors. The methodology is not simple and is difficult to quantitate; however, it is useful qualitatively.

Although multiple other MRS-based approaches have been explored, the other most widely used approach is P-31 MRS, which can determine levels of various phosphorus-containing compounds such as phosphocreatine and ATP. This approach can be used to identify regions of decreased aerobic glycolysis, which are likely hypoxic. In addition the peak position of inorganic phosphate can be used to estimate pH, which is lower in areas of hypoxia.

There are multiple other approaches for assessing hypoxia using MRS, including several types of MR imageable tracers. A recent good review of the subject is by McIntyre.

9.3 Electron Paramagnetic Resonance (EPR)

EPR is similar to nuclear magnetic resonance, but instead of the detection of magnetic nuclei, it detects molecules with unpaired electrons, such as free radicals and transition metal complexes. Paramagnetic tracers such as triarylmethyl (TAM), which show spectral broadening in proportion to the local oxygen concentration have been used for hypoxia imaging. Because the signal level from unpaired electrons is far higher than from nuclei, the magnetic field used is much lower, around 10 mT. The methodology has been evolving in recent years. Currently it is feasible to achieve spatial resolution of 2 mm³ and pO₂ resolution of 3 mmHg over a range of 0–35 mmHg in mice. Time points can be obtained at 3 minute intervals. This method seems to be particularly attractive for looking at temporal changes in hypoxia in-vivo. Commercial systems are not available yet.

9.4 Radiolabeled Tracers for Detection of Hypoxia

Several radio-labeled imaging agents that show increased uptake into hypoxic tissue have been studied for several years, but have not been used clinically. Most of these agents are based on the nitroimidazole structure. Four of the nitroimadazoles are shown in Figure 9.1. All of these have been studied in humans.

Nitroimadazole metabolism is illustrated in Figure 9.2. In hypoxic tissue, following 2-electron reduction the molecule binds to nearby macromolecules. Then time must be allowed to elapse to permit the washout of the agent from well-oxygenated tissue, leaving the bound molecules behind in the hypoxic tissue. All of these agents bind at the same level of hypoxia (pO₂ < 1 mmHg). Attempts to change the binding level by altering the side groups have not been successful. The target-to-background level is similar for all the nitroimadazoles. With fluoromisonidazole a lesion-to-blood ratio of greater than 1.2 is considered hypoxic. Accordingly, the images of these agents do not usually show high contrast and must be assessed quantitatively. The images are often presented in color to be able to roughly determine the tissue-to-blood ratio by inspection. The most significant difference between these agents is that their octanol-water partition coefficients are all different. These differences in lipophylicity strongly affect the rate of tissue wash-in and wash-out. Agents with higher partition coefficients wash in and out more slowly.

Most of the agents listed in Table 9.1 are labeled with Fluorine-18. Because of the relatively long half-life it is feasible to image at 2–4 hours after injection. The target to background ratio steadily improves at later times. One interesting exception to the F-18 agents is pimonidazole. It has been used as a gold standard in animal studies using C-14 pimonidazole and autoradiography. It can also be quantitatively assessed in tissue using immunohistochemistry. It is available commercially under the name "hypoxyprobe." All of these agents have been used in human studies under FDA IND approval.

Another radiolabeled hypoxia imaging agent, developed at Washington University is radioactive copper labeled ATSM, diacetyl-bis(N4-methylthiosemicarbazone). ATSM is a lipophilic molecule that becomes trapped because it becomes negatively charged in a hypoxic environment. There are four isotopes of copper that have been used with ATSM, Cu-60 (t1/2 = 0.40 h), Cu-61 (t1/2 = 3.32 h), Cu-62 (t1/2 = 0.16 h), Cu-64 (t1/2 = 12.7 h). The last one, Cu-64, has been used most widely, because of its longer half life. The literature on ATSM has been somewhat variable with some studies showing good correlation with FMISO, when imaged as early as two hours after injection, while others have found poor

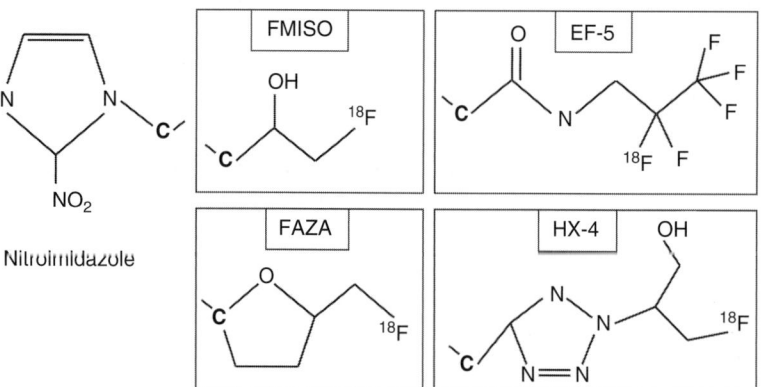

Figure 9.1 All the nitroimadazole imaging agents have a nitroimadazole group, which is connected via the "C" carbon atom to the various structures shown on the right.

Table 9.1 List of hypoxia agents

Full name	Abbreviation	Octanol/Water partition coefficient
Fluoromisonidazole	FMISO	0.44
Fluoroazomycin arabinoside	FAZA	1.1
2-(2-nitro-1H-imidazol-1-yl)-N-(2,2,3,3,3-pentafluoropropyl) acetamide	EF-5	5.7
3-[F]fluoro-2-(4-((2-nitro-1H-imidazol-1-yl) methyl)-1H-1,2,3-triazol-1-yl)propan-1-ol	HX-4	0.2
Pimonidazole	Hypoxyprobe™	8.7

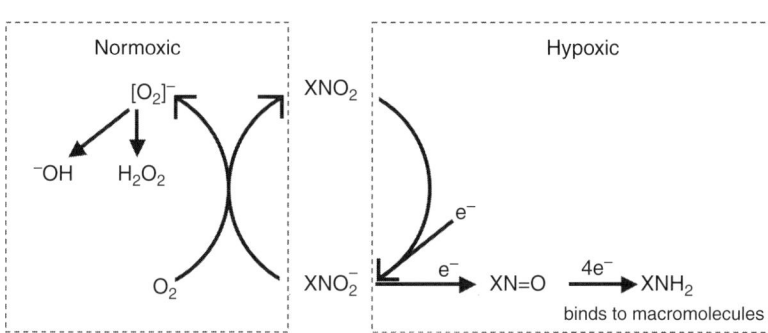

Figure 9.2 Nitroimadazole metabolism. In a well-oxygenated environment the nitroimadazole molecule (XNO_2) is cyclically reduced and oxidized. In a hypoxic environment, additional reduction occurs, resulting in the production of a highly efficient alkylating agent (XNH_2), which binds to macromolecules and is retained by the cell.

correlation on early images with much better correlation on delayed images, as late as sixteen hours after injection.

If hypoxic tumors could be reliably identified, there are a number of ways this information could be used clinically:

1. *Additional radiation could be directed to hypoxic tumors.* Although this is an attractive approach, it is limited in that the radiation dose can be increased only by 50 percent at the most. Another potential problem is that the pattern of hypoxia is not constant, but can shift significantly from day to day.

2. *Re-oxygenation strategies could be investigated, and if shown to be successful, could be used in conjunction with radiotherapy to increase the efficacy of the radiation.* For decades radiotherapists have tried a variety of methods to improve the oxygenation of tumors and thus improve their radiosensitivity. The most commonly used approach is the combination of nicotinamide, a vasodilator, and carbogen, a gas mixture of 95 percent oxygen and 5 percent carbon dioxide. Remarkably, it appears no one has used hypoxia imaging to select patients who might benefit or to monitor changes in hypoxia during reoxygenation.

3. *Hypoxic imaging could be used to identify patients who would benefit from the administration of hypoxic radiosensitizers (HRS) along with the radiotherapy.* One of the first agents studied as a possible HRS was misonidazole. Subsequently several other agents have been studied and have showed significant promise. The largest trial of a HRS was a study of tirapazamine in head and neck cancer, which showed no significant effect, although patients were not stratified by hypoxic status. More recently other agents have been developed that show promise, such as nimorazole and sanazole. This would seem to be an ideal application for hypoxic imaging to select subjects for the trial and later, once an agent was approved, to select patients to receive HRS along with their radiotherapy.

Further Reading

Daşu A, Denekamp J. New insights into factors influencing the clinically relevant oxygen enhancement ratio. *Radiother Oncol.* 1998 Mar;46(3):269–77.

Griffiths JR, Robinson SP. The OxyLite: a fibre-optic oxygen sensor. *Br J Radiol.* 1999 Jul;72(859):627–30.

Kaanders JH, Bussink J, van der Kogel AJ. ARCON: a novel biology-based approach in radiotherapy. *Lancet Oncol.* 2002 Dec;3(12):728–37.

Kizaka-Kondoh S, Konse-Nagasawa H. Significance of nitroimidazole compounds and hypoxia-inducible factor-1 for imaging tumor hypoxia. *Cancer Sci.* 2009 Aug;100(8):1366–73.

Krishna MC, Matsumoto S, Yasui H, Saito K, Devasahayam N, Subramanian S, Mitchell JB. Electron paramagnetic resonance imaging of tumor pO2. *Radiat Res.* 2012 Apr;177(4):376–86.

Krohn KA, Link JM, Mason RP. Molecular imaging of hypoxia. *J Nucl Med.* 2008 Jun;49 Suppl 2:129S–48S.

Laurent F, Benard P, Canal P, Soula G. Autoradiographic distribution of [14C]-labelled pimonidazole in rhabdomyosarcoma-bearing rats and pigmented mice. *Cancer Chemother Pharmacol.* 1988;22(4):308–15.

Lin Z, Mechalakos J, Nehmeh S, Schoder H, Lee N, Humm J, Ling CC. The influence of changes in tumor hypoxia on dose-painting treatment plans based on 18F-FMISO PET. *Int J Radiat Oncol Biol Phys.* 2008 Mar 15;70(4):1219–28.

McIntyre DJ, Madhu B, Lee SH, Griffiths JR. Magnetic resonance spectroscopy of cancer metabolism and response to therapy. *Radiat Res.* 2012 Apr;177(4):398–435.

Mees G, Dierckx R, Vangestel C, Van de Wiele C. Molecular imaging of hypoxia with radiolabelled agents. *Eur J Nucl Med Mol Imaging.* 2009 Oct;36(10):1674–86.

Stone HB, Brown JM, Phillips TL, Sutherland RM. Oxygen in human tumors: correlations between methods of measurement and response to therapy. Summary of a workshop held November 19–20, 1992, at the National Cancer Institute, Bethesda, Maryland. *Radiat Res.* 1993 Dec;136(3):422–34.

Sugie C, Shibamoto Y, Ito M, Ogino H, Suzuki H, Uto Y, Nagasawa H, Hori H. Reevaluation of the radiosensitizing effects of sanazole and nimorazole in vitro and in vivo. *J Radiat Res.* 2005 Dec;46(4):453–9.

Receptor Imaging

Michael Graham

Cell surface receptors and their associated receptor ligands are fundamental and essential aspects of the physiology and homeostasis of virtually all multicellular organisms. In addition, many tumors have either unique receptors or have significantly up-regulated receptors that can be exploited for both diagnosis and therapy. There are currently several approved radiopharmaceuticals that are available, as well as a major amount of research going into the development of new receptor-based imaging agents. The currently available agents are listed in Table 10.1.

The obvious key approach for receptor imaging is to identify a ligand that binds to the receptor and that can be imaged. This usually involves an imaging entity, a linker, and the binding ligand, see Figure 10.1.

There are several considerations that must be taken into account in the selection of specific ligands, linkers, and labels for different situations. Some of the most important general considerations in selecting a specific combination are metabolic stability, in-vivo pharmacokinetics, and imaging label characteristics. The combined imaging agent must be metabolically stable, so that the label remains attached to the ligand. The ligand should have high receptor specificity and affinity, so that it binds to the desired receptor well and does not bind significantly elsewhere. The label should have a half-life that is compatible with the rate that the ligand binds to the receptor and clears from the background. Other considerations are discussed in the pages that follow.

10.1 Receptor Ligands

10.1.1 Oligopeptide Ligands

Since every receptor has to have a binding ligand, the most direct approach is to identify the endogenous or exogenous binding protein and use it in the design of a receptor imaging agent. Generally, this direct approach is not successful because of the relatively rapid metabolic degradation of endogenous ligands. For instance, somatostatin has a half-life in the circulation of only 2–3 minutes. The usual approach is to modify the endogenous ligand to decrease or block its metabolism, but at the same time preserve the receptor affinity. This approach has been used successfully for the somatostatin receptor, which can be imaged with In-111 pentetreotide. The label is In-111, the linker is di-ethylene-triamine-penta-acetic (DTPA), and the ligand is an oligopeptide consisting of eight amino acids similar to the binding part of somatostatin.

Other oligopeptide receptor ligand analogs that have been labeled for imaging include cholecystokinin, gastrin, bombesin, bradykinin, melanocortin, and angiotensin. A three amino acid oligopeptide of particular interest is the arginine-glycine-aspartate peptide (RGD), which binds to the alpha5-beta3 integrin and is a marker of neoangiogenesis.

10.1.2 Antibodies

An antibody will bind very effectively to a specific antigen, which can be selected to bind to a specific receptor. One of the best known examples is capromab pendetide, which binds to prostate specific membrane antigen (PSMA). The label is In-111, the linker is pendetide (a derivative of DTPA), and the ligand is a mouse monoclonal antibody selected to bind to PSMA. Antibodies are produced by immunizing mice to the desired antigen and by selecting the cells from the mouse spleen that show the best binding characteristics. Once the right cells have been identified they can be fused with mouse myeloma cells, which can be grown and large amounts of the antibody can be produced. This approach has been very successfully employed leading to the development of a large number of useful antibodies.

Table 10.1 Imaging Agents and Their Targets

Imaging agent	Receptor target	Tissue target
In-111 pentetreotide	Somatostatin receptor	Neuroendocrine tumors
I-123 meta-iodobenzylguanidine	Norepinephrine re-uptake	Neuroblastoma
In-111 capromab pendetide	Prostate-specific membrane antigen	Prostate cancer
Y-90 ibritumomab tiuxetan	CD-20 on lymphocytes	Lymphoma therapy
I-131 tositumomab	CD-20 on lymphocytes	Lymphoma therapy
I-123 ioflupane	Dopamine transporter	Parkinson's disease
F-18 florbetapir	Beta-amyloid	Alzheimer's dementia

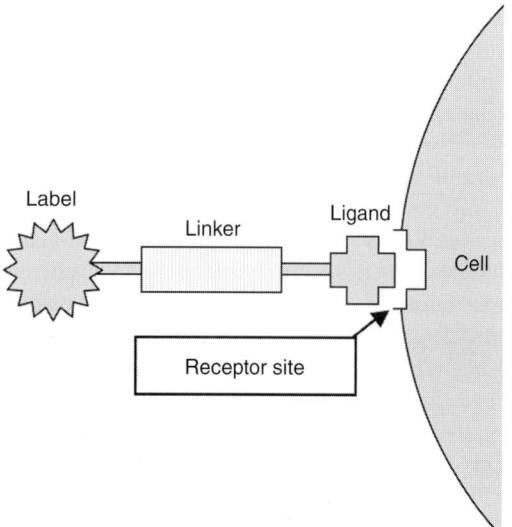

Figure 10.1 A receptor imaging agent consists of an imaging entity (radioactive atom, fluorophor, iron oxide, etc), a linker (DTPA, DOTA, etc.), and a receptor binding ligand.

Two significant limitations of using antibodies for receptor imaging are the slow clearance, typically several days for intact antibodies, and their slow diffusion out of the circulation, due to their large molecular weight. Multiple approaches have been undertaken to address these problems, primarily by using lower molecular weight fragments of the antibodies that still retain their binding characteristics but are cleared more rapidly than the intact antibody. These include Fab fragments, diabodies, and minibodies.

10.1.3 Aptamers

Aptamers are DNA and RNA sequences that can fold into a wide variety of three-dimensional shapes. By starting with a very large number of sequences ($\sim 10^{13}$), it is possible to identify a specific sequence that avidly binds to a selected target, such as a receptor. Although this approach has been recognized for over twenty years, only recently is it beginning to be used to create binding ligands for receptor imaging.

The advantages of aptamers include high binding affinity, high binding specificity, stable structure, small size, little immunogenicity and ease of synthesis. When used in-vivo the aptamers have to be protected, typically by attachment of polyethylene glycol (PEG) polymer chains to the aptamer (PEGylation). Otherwise the aptamers are cleared very rapidly from the circulation. Examples of aptamer-targeted receptors for in-vivo imaging include elastase for inflammation, thrombin for thrombus imaging, and tenascin-C and PSMA for tumor imaging. Although no aptamers have yet been approved for human administration, this is a very promising approach that will likely yield some very useful agents in the future.

10.1.4 Small Molecules

The major advantage of using small molecules is that the pharmacokinetics, in general, are more rapid than for larger molecules, such as oligopeptides or antibodies. The small molecules that have been identified are either an analog of an endogenous molecule that is known to interact with the receptor, for example norepinephrine uptake receptor (meta-iodobenzylguanidine), or those identified through screening a large number of compounds with structures similar to the endogenous receptor ligand. An example of the second approach is a set of small molecule ligands that bind to the oxytocin receptor. The goals in selecting a small molecule receptor ligand is high affinity for the receptor, high specificity (minimal binding to other receptor or tissues), minimal metabolic degradation, minimal immunogenicity and relative ease of synthesis.

10.1.5 Quantitative Characterization of Receptor Ligands

Common terms used to describe receptor binding ligands are: affinity, specificity, and receptor density. Qualitatively, the meaning of these terms are: affinity is how tightly the ligand binds to the receptor; specificity is how well it binds to the receptor compared to other receptors and tissues; receptor density is how many receptors there are per unit area of cell surface.

By measuring the time-dependent uptake of the labeled receptor ligand into tissue, along with measurement of the activity in plasma or in a reference tissue, it is possible to determine specific binding parameters in order to characterize the binding of the ligand to tissue in-vivo. This information is essential for comparing the behavior of different ligands and in understanding the meaning of the ligand uptake into tissues of interest.

Most of the parameters listed here are determined in-vitro or in-vivo using PET imaging. These parameters are particularly important in comparing different ligands and in identifying the most promising for in-vivo studies.

Receptor density (Bmax) is the amount of drug required to saturate a population of receptors and is a measure of the number of receptors present in a tissue. It is often derived in-vitro using the Scatchard plot.

Equilibrium dissociation constant (K_d) is inversely related to the affinity of receptor binding. It is defined as K_{off}/K_{on}. K_{on} and K_{off} are the rate constants for attaching to and detaching from a receptor. It is roughly equal to $\underline{IC_{50}}$, which is the concentration of a reference ligand required to inhibit 50 percent of ligand binding to the receptor of interest. An example would be the effect of somatostatin on the binding of octreotide to one of the somatostatin receptor subtypes (SST). The IC50 for octreotide for SST2 is 2.0 nM, while the IC50 for SST3 is 187 nM. This means that the affinity for SST2 is much higher than for SST3. The difference between K_d and IC_{50} is covered in Krohn and Link.

Binding potential (BP) is a combined measure of the density of available receptors and the affinity of a drug to the receptor. It is defined as B_{max}/K_d, or approximately as the ratio at equilibrium of the concentration of specifically bound ligand in tissue to the concentration of free ligand in tissue. There are a number of subtly different versions of BP, which are discussed by Innis. It is a widely used parameter because it is relatively easy to measure with PET imaging and is an approximate measure of receptor density.

Volume of distribution is another practical way of roughly quantitating receptor density. Volume of distribution is defined as the amount of tracer injected divided by the equilibrium concentration in the plasma. The approach has been widely used in physiology and medicine to measure various physiologic volumes such as the plasma volume, using labeled albumin as the tracer. With receptors the volume of distribution is the concentration within a tissue divided by the concentration in plasma. The resulting calculated volume of distribution is usually far larger than the plasma volume and does not represent any real physiologic volume. A large volume of distribution represents a high receptor density in a tissue. Another way to roughly determine the volume of distribution is to compare uptake in a target tissue to uptake in a reference tissue known to contain no receptors. In brain studies, this is often the cerebellum.

Further Reading

Bigott-Hennkens HM, Dannoon S, Lewis MR, Jurisson SS. In vitro receptor binding assays: general methods and considerations. *Q J Nucl Med Mol Imaging*. 2008 Sep;52(3):245–53.

Ellington AD, Szostak JW. In vitro selection of RNA molecules that bind specific ligands. *Nature*. 1990 Aug 30;346(6287):818–22.

Innis RB, Cunningham VJ, Delforge J, Fujita M, Gjedde A, Gunn RN, et al. Consensus nomenclature for in vivo imaging of reversibly binding radioligands. *J Cereb Blood Flow Metab*. 2007 Sep;27(9):1533–9.

Krohn KA, Link JM. Interpreting enzyme and receptor kinetics: keeping it simple, but not too simple. *Nucl Med Biol*. 2003 Nov;30(8):819–26.

Mankoff DA, Link JM, Linden HM, Sundararajan L, Krohn KA. Tumor receptor imaging. *J Nucl Med*. 2008 Jun;49 Suppl 2:149S–63S.

Mohanty C, Das M, Kanwar JR, Sahoo SK. Receptor mediated tumor targeting: an emerging approach for cancer therapy. *Curr Drug Deliv*. 2011 Jan;8(1):45–58.

Olafsen T, Betting D, Kenanova VE, Salazar FB, Clarke P, Said J, et al. Recombinant anti-CD20 antibody fragments for small-animal PET imaging of B-cell lymphomas. *J Nucl Med*. 2009 Sep;50(9):1500–8.

Pool SE, Krenning EP, Koning GA, van Eijck CH, Teunissen JJ, Kam B, et al. Preclinical and clinical studies of peptide receptor radionuclide therapy. *Semin Nucl Med*. 2010 May;40(3):209–18.

Smith AL, Freeman SM, Stehouwer JS, Inoue K, Voll RJ, Young LJ, et al. Synthesis and evaluation of C-11, F-18 and I-125 small molecule radioligands for detecting oxytocin receptors. *Bioorg Med Chem*. 2012 Apr 15;20(8):2721–38.

Soontornworajit B, Wang Y. Nucleic acid aptamers for clinical diagnosis: cell detection and molecular imaging. *Anal Bioanal Chem*. 2011 Feb;399(4):1591–9.

Apoptosis

Heather Jacene

11.1 The Apoptosis Cellular Pathway

Apoptosis is the process of programmed cell death and is critical for growth and development and the maintenance of cellular homeostasis. Cells committed to death through the apoptotic pathway are dissembled according to a coordinated sequence of events. The classic morphologic changes during apoptosis are loss of communication and detachment from neighboring cells, condensation of chromatin at the nuclear membrane, fragmentation of the nuclear membrane, cell shrinkage, and formation of apoptotic bodies which are subsequently phagocytosed. Apoptosis is energy dependent and a distinct feature is that the cell's plasma membrane remains intact. There is no accompanying inflammatory response and no evidence of the cell's previous existence. In contrast, cellular necrosis is a disorderly process which results in surrounding inflammation and oftentimes residual tissue scarring.

Apoptosis is mediated through a number of cellular proteins and signaling pathways (Figure 11.1). The major family of proteins responsible for apoptosis is cysteine proteases called caspases. Caspases are inactivated in the cell cytoplasm (as procaspases) until receiving a death signal. Once activated, initiator caspases activate effector caspases which in turn activate the rest of the machinery needed for programmed cell death. Activation of the initiator caspases occurs via the intrinsic or mitochondrial pathway or via the extrinsic pathway.

The intrinsic (mitochondrial) pathway is induced by cellular stress or the loss of survival signals. Upon receiving such signals, mitochondria release cytochrome c through pores in the mitochondrial membrane causing apoptosome formation through oligomerization of molecules, Apaf-1 in vertebrates. Apoptosome formation results in activation of initiator caspases. The Bcl-2 family of proteins regulates the mitochondrial pathway through both anti-apoptotic

(e.g., Bcl-2) and pro-apoptotic (e.g., Bak, Bax) properties.

The extrinsic pathway is activated by the binding of death ligands (e.g., tumor necrosis factor alpha) to the extracellular component of death receptors in the cell membrane. This results in the recruitment of adaptor molecules which activate initiator caspases. Subsquent formation of death receptor signaling complexes activates effector caspases leading to apoptosis. An immune response or tumorigenesis can initiate the extrinsic pathway.

11.2 Agents for Molecular Imaging of Apoptosis

Large proteins, small peptides, and organic molecules have been designed for imaging different targets in the apoptosis pathway (Table 11.1). The first and most widely studied is Annexin V radiolabeled with technetium-99m (^{99m}Tc) and a new promising agent is fluorine-18 (^{18}F) labeled 5-fluoropentyl-2-methyl-malonic acid (^{18}F-ML-10) for positron emission tomography (PET). The other agents listed in Table 11.1 have also been shown to detect apoptosis in preclinical models and are reviewed in detail by De Saint-Hubert and Reshef et al.

11.2.1 Annexin V

Annexin V is an endogenous human protein that targets phosphatidylserine (PS). In non-apoptotic cells, PS is found on the inner layer of the cell membrane. As one of the first events of apoptosis, PS translocates to the outer layer of the cell membrane (Figure 11.2). Annexin V has been radiolabeled with a variety of radioisotopes (Table 11.1) as well as magnetic nanoparticles and gadolinium-containing liposomes for magnetic resonance imaging (MRI) and fluorescent markers for optical imaging.

As stated, the most studied agent is ^{99m}Tc-Annexin and its safety in humans and biodistribution are

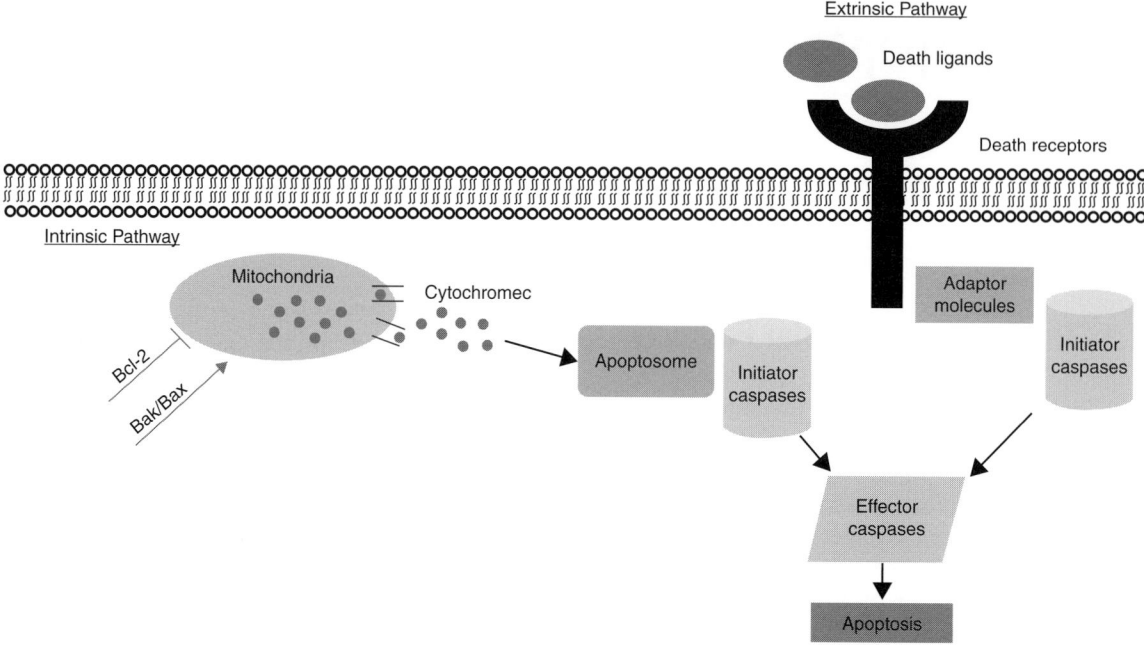

Figure 11.1 The apoptotic pathway.

Table 11.1 Molecular Imaging Agents for Apoptosis

Probe	Target	Radioisotopes and non-radioactive labels
Annexin V	Phosphatidylserine	^{99m}Tc, ^{111}In, ^{123}I, ^{125}I, ^{18}F, ^{68}Ga, ^{64}Cu, ^{124}I, magnetic nanoparticles, fluorescent markers
C2 doman of synaptotagmin	Phosphatidylserine	^{99m}Tc, magnetic nanoparticles
Duramycin	Phosphatidylethanolamine	^{99m}Tc
Isatin	Caspase-3	^{18}F, ^{11}C
5-fluoropentyl-2-methyl-malionic acid	Plasma membrane depolarization	^{18}F
Fluorobenzyl triphenlphosphonium	Mitrocohondrial membrane potential	^{18}F

^{99m}Tc: technetium-99m; ^{111}In: indium-111; ^{123}I: iodine-123; ^{125}I: iodine-125; ^{18}F: fluorine-18; ^{68}Ga: gallium-68, ^{64}Cu: copper-64; ^{124}I: iodine-124; ^{11}C: choline-11

established. The normal biodistribution of ^{99m}Tc-Annexin V, using a hydrazinonicotinamide (HYNIC) linker molecule for radiolabeling, is high uptake in the kidneys and liver and moderate uptake in the spleen and red marrow (Figure 11.3). The primary route of ^{99m}Tc-HYNIC-Annexin excretion is renal. Investigations of ^{18}F-Annexin V have shown lesser uptake in the kidneys, liver, and spleen.

The major limitation of imaging apoptosis with Annexin V is specificity between apoptotic and necrotic cell death. PS on the inner layer of the cell membrane is also exposed during necrosis once the cell membrane ruptures. Annexin V imaging is also limited by low target-to-background ratios due to the large size of the protein and subsequent slower clearance from background tissues, despite relatively fast clearance from the blood pool.

11.2.2 Radiolabeled Small Molecules

Given the inability of Annexin V to distinguish between apoptosis and necrosis, imaging agents targeting more specific molecules and events in the apoptotic pathway, including caspase activation and

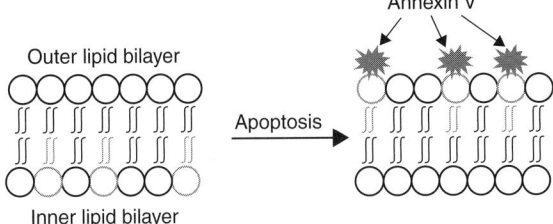

Figure 11.2 Translocation of phosphatidylserine (light gray) from the inner to outer layer of the cell membrane during apoptosis makes it a good target for Annexin V.

alterations of the mitochondrial membrane with preserved integrity, are being developed.

Small-molecule caspase inhibitors have been radiolabeled with ^{18}F and choline-11 (^{11}C) and have been shown to have a high affinity for caspase 3, an effector caspase common to both the intrinsic and extrinsic pathways. These agents, however, have been tested in just a few preclinical models.

^{18}F-ML-10 is one of a group of novel small-molecule compounds (Aposense compounds, Aposense Ltd, Israel) designed to detect alterations of the mitochondrial membrane in cells undergoing apoptosis. In vitro studies have demonstrated selective uptake of ^{18}F-ML-10 in apoptotic, but not necrotic, cells. Preclinical models demonstrated rapid clearance of ^{18}F-ML-10 with no significant tracer uptake in major organs, leading to potentially high target-to-background ratios. This agent is currently undergoing evaluations in clinical trials.

11.3 Clinical Applications for Apoptosis Imaging

11.3.1 Cardiology

Apoptosis has been shown to have a role in the pathophysiology of atherosclerotic plaque rupture, myocardial infarction/reperfusion injury, myocarditis, drug-induced cardiotoxicity, cardiomyopathy, cardiac transplant rejection, and chronic heart failure. For example, myocardiocyte death is mediated by apoptosis in the first hours after an ischemic event or reperfusion injuries prior to the onset of cellular necrosis. Molecular imaging of apoptosis provides insight into the biology of cardiac diseases, and studies have shown that the apoptotic pathway is typically activated and can be detected prior to currently available cardiac biomarkers. Molecular imaging of apoptosis has the

potential to be used for risk stratification, tailoring of therapeutic approaches (e.g. guiding intervention after myocardial infarction) and monitoring response to therapy.

11.3.2 Neurology

Cerebral stroke is another model used to evaluate apoptosis imaging agents. Visualization of apoptosis with ^{18}F-ML-10 has been demonstrated in a human study of patients with acute cerebral stroke. A potential limitation of apoptosis imaging in the brain is nonspecific accumulation of the imaging agent due to disruption of the blood–brain barrier; however, this is not a unique limitation and should be considered for any brain imaging probe.

11.3.3 Oncology

Apoptosis is an important pathway in cancer because the increased number of cells in tumors may be due to increased cell proliferation or decreased cell death. Oncogenes that inhibit apoptosis have been identified and often loss of function of these oncogenes leads to tumorigenesis. For example, mutations in the Bcl-2 gene have been demonstrated in most follicular lymphomas. Loss of apoptosis has also been shown to be important for the metastatic spread of tumor.

Prior to therapy, accumulation of ^{99m}Tc-HYNIC-annexin has been shown to correlate with the number of apoptotic cells by histopathology in head and neck cancer, although in other clinical studies and tumor types baseline uptake was variable. Imaging apoptosis prior to treatment could guide therapy and potentially provide prognostic information. This is because the mechanism of cell death of different tumor types in response to therapy varies. Tumors that respond to low-doses of radiation, such as lymphoma, are more susceptible to the induction of apoptosis, compared to those tumors requiring higher doses or those that are radio-resistant.

There is also great interest in imaging apoptosis as a biomarker of response to therapy. In addition to radiotherapy, many chemotherapy agents also induce apoptosis. Apoptosis occurs early (within hours to days) after successful therapy and in oncology clinical studies, post-treatment scans were typically performed within three days after the completion of therapy.

Early clinical studies in patients with non-small cell lung cancer, squamous cell head and neck cancer, breast cancer and lymphoma have shown correlations

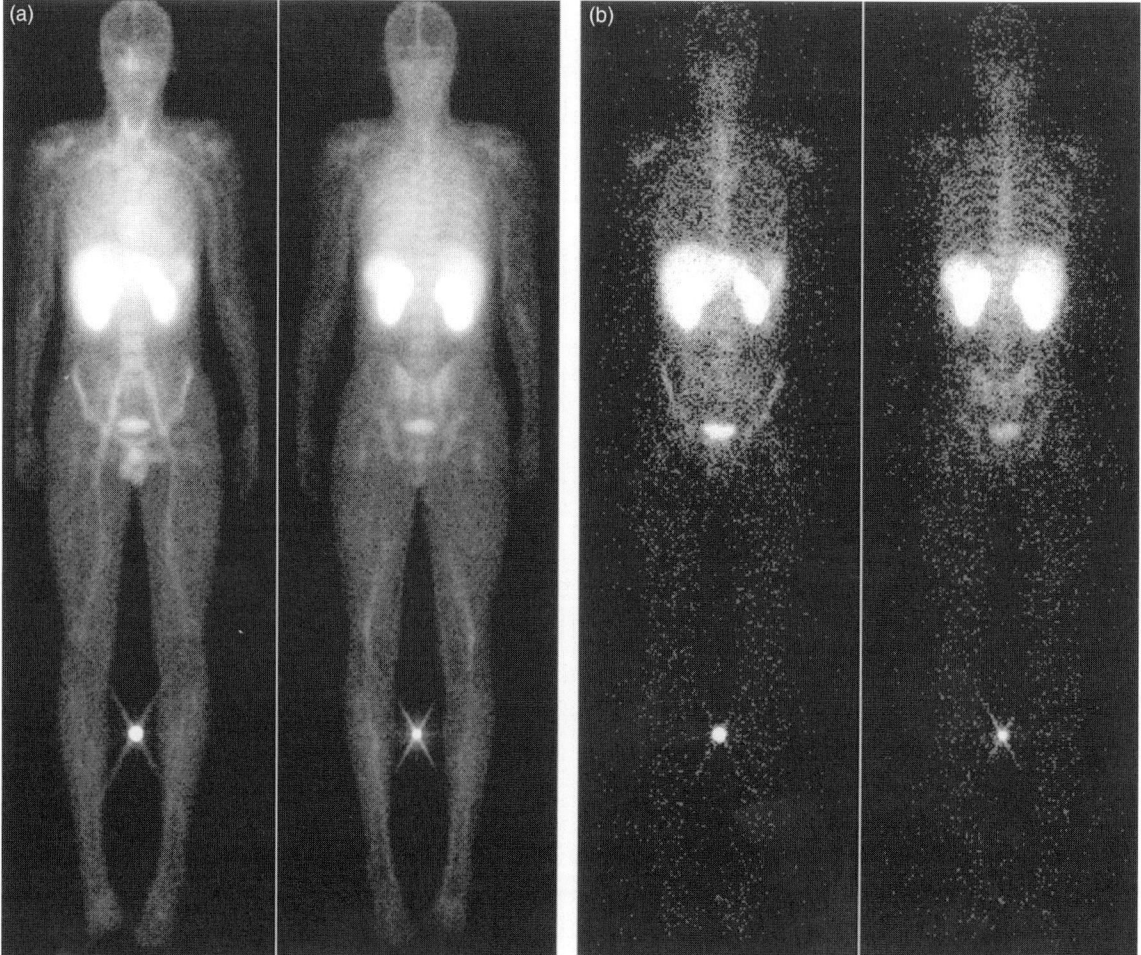

Figure 11.3 Normal biodistribution of ^{99m}Tc-HYNIC-Annexin V. This research was originally published in JNM. Kemerink GJ, Liu X, Kieffer D, et al. Safety, Biodistribution, and Dosimetry of ^{99m}Tc-HYNIC-Annexin V, a Novel Human Recombinant Annexin V for Human Application. *J Nucl Med*. 2003;44(6):947–952. Figure 11.3© by the Society of Nuclear Medicine and Molecular Imaging, Inc. Reprinted with Permission.

between changes in ^{99m}Tc-HYNIC-annexin tumor uptake between pre-treatment and early post-treatment scans and outcome. Increases in ^{99m}Tc-HYNIC-annexin tumor uptake were seen in those who responded to therapy, while those with progression had no increase or a decrease in uptake. ^{18}F-ML-10 also predicted response on MRI 2 months after whole brain radiation in patients with brain metastases. These results are very encouraging and more and larger studies are needed.

Further Reading

Belhocine T, Steinmetz N, Hustinx R, Bartsch P, Jerusalem G, Seidel L, Rigo P, Green A. Increased uptake of the apoptosis-imaging agent (99m)Tc recombinant human Annexin V in human tumors after one course of chemotherapy as a predictor of tumor response and patient prognosis. *Clin Cancer Res* 2002;8:2766–2774.

Blankenberg FG. In vivo detection of apoptosis. *J Nucl Med* 2008;49:81S–95S.

Cohen A, Shirvan A, Levin G, Grimberg H, Reshef A, Ziv I. From the Gla domain to a novel small-molecule detector of apoptosis. *Cell Res* 2009;19:625–637.

De Saint-Hubert M. Bauwens M, Verbruggen A, Mottaghy FM. Apoptosis imaging to monitor cancer therapy: the road to fast treatment evaluation? *Current Pharmaceutical Biotechnology* 2012;13:571–583.

Haas RL, de Jong D, Valdés Olmos RA, Hoefnagel CA, van den Heuvel I, Zerp SF, Bartelink H, Verheij M. In vivo imaging of radiation-induced apoptosis in follicular lymphoma patients. *Int J Radiat Oncol Biol Phys* 2004;59:782–787.

Hu S, Kiesewetter DO, Zhu L, Guo N, Gao H, Liu G, Hida N, Lang L, Niu G, Chen X. Longitudinal PET imaging of doxorubicin-induced cell death with (18) F-Annexin V. *Mol Imaging Biol* 2012 Mar 6. [Epub ahead of print].

Kartachova M, van Zandwijk N, Burgers S, van Tinteren H, Verheij, Valdés Olmos RA. Prognostic significance of ^{99m}Tc-HYNIC-rh-Annexin V scintigraphy during platinum-based chemotherapy in advanced lung cancer. *J Clin Oncol* 2007;25:2534–2539.

Kemerink GJ, Liu X, Kieffer D, Ceyssens S, Mortelmans L, Verbruggen AM, Steinmetz ND, Vanderheyden JL, Green AM, Verbeke K. Safety, biodistribution, and dosimetry of 99mTc-HYNIC-Annexin V, a novel human recombinant Annexin V for human application. *J Nucl Med* 2003;44:947–952.

Korngold EC, Jaffer FA, Wiessleder R, Sosnovik DE. Noninvasive imaging of apoptosis in cardiovascular disease. *Heart Fail Rev* 2008;13:163–173.

Munõz-Pinedo C. Signaling pathways that regulate life and cell death: evolution of apoptosis in the context of self-defense. *Adv Exp Med Biol* 2012;738:124–143.

Reshef A, Shirvan A, Akselrod-Ballin A, Wall A, ZIv, I. Small-molecule biomarkers for clinical PET imaging of apoptosis. *J Nucl Med* 2010;51:837–840.

van de Wiele C, Lahorte C, Vermeersch H, Loose D, Mervillie K, Steinmetz ND, Vanderheyden JL, Cuvelier CA, Slegers G, Dierck RA. Quantitative tumor apoptosis imaging using technetium-99m-HYNIC-Annexin V single photon emission computed tomography. *J Clin Oncol* 2003;21:3483–3487.

Verheij M. Clinical biomarkers and imaging for radiotherapy-induced cell death. *Cancer Metastasis Rev* 2008;27:471–480.

Chapter 12

Angiogenesis

Hossein Jadvar

Angiogenesis plays an important role both physiologically and pathologically and relates to the process of hypoxia-induced formation of new blood vessels from preexisting vessels. It can be useful in some conditions such as collateralization in ischemic myocardium but it is also associated with pathologic conditions such as chronic inflammatory diseases, age-related macular degeneration, and cancer. Tumor growth beyond 1–2 mm is angiogenesis-dependent, which is induced by complex multistep interactions between the tumor and the host (angiogenic switch). Inhibition of angiogenesis may inhibit tumor growth (cytostatic rather than cytotoxic). Early anti-angiogenesis treatment strategies generally resulted in disappointing results which may have been due to flaws in clinical trial design and choice of outcome measures. However, a new generation of anti-angiogenic agents has shown promising results in combination with chemoradiation therapy.

Imaging angiogenesis is critical for the timing of anti-angiogenesis therapy and for the assessment of therapy efficacy. Angiogenesis is a complex biological process and is regulated by abundant molecular pathways including, but not limited to, vascular endothelial growth factor (VEGF), integrins, and metalloproteinases (MMPs). All major imaging modalities (optical imaging, ultrasound, computed tomography, magnetic resonance imaging, single photon emission computed tomography, positron emission tomography) may be employed for imaging some particular feature of angiogenesis indirectly (e.g. perfusion) or directly (e.g. targeted to biologically relevant molecules).

Ultrasound may be used with nontargeted or targeted (to angiogenic markers) microbubble contrast agents for assessment of tumor vascularity and monitoring response to treatment. It is a widely available, relatively low-cost imaging modality that allows portable real-time imaging without ionizing radiation. Computed tomography (CT) with iodinated contrast agents may be employed to assess vascular enhancement over time and diffusion of the contrast material into the extravascular interstitial space. The tissue distribution of contrast material may be modeled to measure such parameters as tissue blood flow, blood volume, and capillary permeability surface area. Magnetic resonance imaging (MRI) provides excellent soft tissue contrast without ionizing radiation. Arterial spin labeling (ASL) and blood oxygenation level-dependent (BOLD) imaging can provide indirect information about vascularity without the use of contrast agents. However, macromolecular contrast material in conjunction with dynamic contrast enhanced (DCE) MRI can be used to assess tumor vascularity and permeability. Research is underway to design and synthesize targeted MR contrast agents that provide direct information about biomarkers involved in angiogenesis such as the VEGF receptor and integrins.

There is a relatively rich literature on the use of scintigraphy with PET and SPECT in imaging various biomarkers in angiogenesis. Perfusion can be imaged quantitatively with ^{15}O-H2O PET although the very short half-life of 2 minutes for ^{15}O limits its use to centers with a cyclotron facility. Radiolabeled VEGF isoforms and anti-VEGF antibodies have also been employed for scintigraphic imaging of angiogenesis.

An important biomarker that has been employed for imaging angiogenesis is the cell adhesion molecule, integrin $\alpha v\beta 3$, which is upregulated on tumoral endothelial cells and some tumor cells. All integrins are α/β heterodimeric glycoproteins. The individual α subunits (18 known subunits) combine with individual β subunits (8 known subunits) to create 24 unique $\alpha\beta$ heterodimers. Several classes of integrins recognize the Arginine-Glycine-Aspartic acid (RGD) sequence present in extracellular matrix (ECM) proteins (e.g. fibronectin, vitronectin, collagen, osteopontin, fibrinogen), allowing integrins to

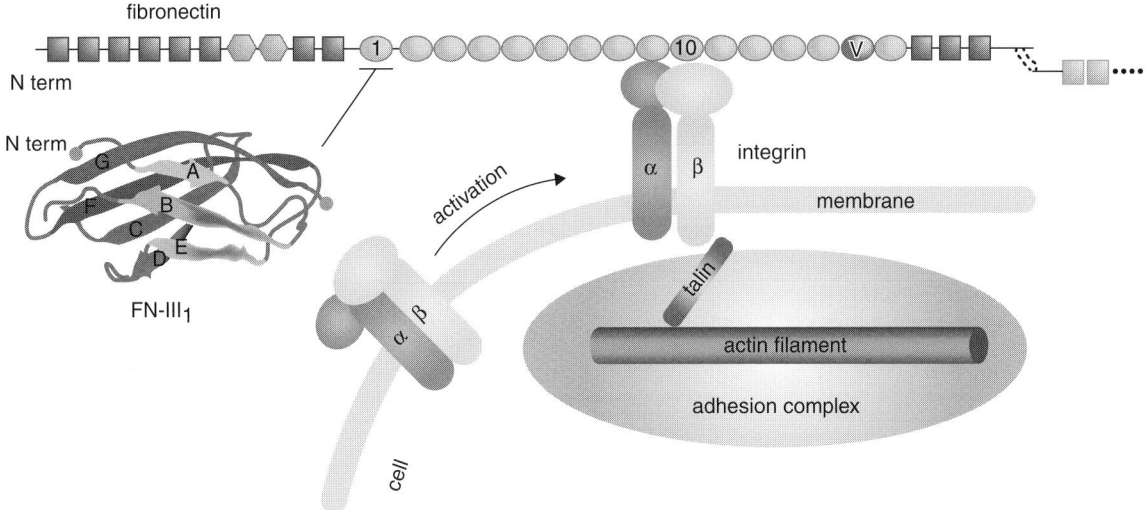

Figure 12.1 Schematic view of integrin-based cell-matrix interaction (From: NIH Resource for Macromolecular Modeling & Bioinformatics, University of Illinois at Urbana-Champaign).

link cytoskeletal proteins with the ECM and other cells and to be involved in bi-directional signaling that alters cellular functions (i.e. cell–cell and cell–matrix interaction and communication) (Figure 12.1). Among these interactions are the adhesion of both endothelial cells and cancer cells to ECM proteins, interactions that are integral to tumor growth, metastasis, and angiogenesis.

There have been a number of radiolabeled RGD peptides that have been synthesized for SPECT or PET imaging of integrin $\alpha v \beta 3$ expression in tumors and monitoring of response to anti-angiogenic drugs such as bevacizumab. For example, ^{18}F-Galacto-RGD has been shown to be useful in imaging integrin expression in cancer. It is interesting to note that the uptake of ^{18}F-Galacto-RGD and FDG may not correlate suggesting that tumor expression of $\alpha v \beta 3$ integrin and glucose metabolism reflect different biological aspects of malignancy. Interested readers are referred to excellent published reviews of preclinical and clinical molecular imaging of angiogenesis with various radiotracers that have been developed and investigated for imaging VEGF/VEGFR, integrins, and matrix metalloproteinases.

Despite relatively extensive research, the exact role of imaging angiogenesis in cancer (and other pathologic conditions) remains unsettled. Further research will clarify how and when imaging tumor angiogenesis can contribute to the holy grail of risk-adapted "personalized/precision" cancer care.

Further Reading

1. Pircher A, Hilbe W, Heidegger I, Drevs J, Tichelli, Medinger M. Biomarkers in tumor angiogenesis and anti-angiogenic therapy. *Int J Mol Sci* 2011; 12:7077–99.

2. Zhu L, Niu G, Fang X, Chen X. Preclinical molecular imaging of tumor angiogenesis. *Q J Nucl Med Mol Imaging* 2010; 54:291–308.

3. Kiessling F, Razansky D, Alves F. Anatomical and microstructural imaging of angiogenesis. *Eur J Nucl Med Mol Imaging* 2010; 37 Suppl 1:S4–19.

4. Naumov GN, Akslen LA, Folkman J. Role of angiogenesis in human tumor dormancy: animal models of the angiogenic switch. *Cell Cycle* 2006; 5:1779–87.

5. Medina MA, Munoz-Chapuli R, Quesada AR. Challenges of antiangiogenic cancer therapy: trials and errors, and renewed hope. *J Cell Mol Med* 2007; 11:374–82.

6. McDonald DM, Choyke PL. Imaging of angiogenesis: from microscope to clinic. *Nat Med* 2003; 9:713–25.

7. Iagaru A, Gambhir SS. Imaging tumor angiogenesis: the road to clinical utility. *AJR Am J Roentgenol* 2013; 201:W183-W191.

8. Zhu L, Niu G, Fang X, Chen X. Preclinical molecular imaging of tumor angiogenesis. *AJR Am J Roentgenol* 2009; 193:304–13.

9. Charnley N, Donalson S, Price P. Imaging angiogenesis. *Methods Mol Biol* 2009; 467:25–51.

10. Cai W, Chen X. Multimodality molecular imaging of tumor angiogenesis. *J Nucl Med* 2008; 49 Suppl 2:113S-28S.

11. Provenzale JM. Imaging of angiogenesis: clinical techniques and novel imaging methods. *AJR Am J Roentgenol* 2007; 188:11–23.

12. Neeman M, Gilad AA, Dafni H, Cohen B. Molecular imaging of angiogenesis. *J Magn Reson Imaging* 2007; 25:1–12.

13. Miller JC, Pien HH, Sahani D, Sorensen AG, Thrall JH. Imaging angiogenesis: applications and potential for drug development. *J Natl Cancer Inst* 2005; 97:172–87.

14. Schirner M, Menrad A, Stephens A, Frenzel T, Hauff P, Licha K. Molecular imaging of tumor angiogenesis. *Ann N Y Acad Sci* 2004; 1014:67–75.

15. Brack SS, Dinkelborg LM, Neri D. Molecular targeting of angiogenesis for imaging and therapy. *Eur J Nucl Med Mol Imaging* 2004; 31:1327–41.

16. Patel N, Harris AL, Gleeson FV, Vallis KA. Clinical imaging of tumor angiogenesis. *Future Oncol* 2012; 81:1443–59.

17. Stacey MR, Maxfield MW, Sinusas AJ. Targeted molecular imaging of angiogenesis in PET and SPECT: a review. *Yale J Biol Med* 2012; 85:75–86.

18. Dikgraaf I, Boeman OC. Radionuclide imaging of tumor angiogenesis. *Cancer Biother Radiopharm* 2009; 24:637–47.

19. Dijkgraaf I, Boerman OC. Molecular imaging of angiogenesis with SPECT. *Eur J Nucl Med Mol Imaging* 2010; 37 Suppl 1:S104–13.

20. Mulder WJ, Strijkers GJ, Nicolay K, Griffioen AW. Quantum dots for multimodal molecular imaging of angiogenesis. *Angiogenesis* 2010; 13:131–4.

21. Snoeks TJ, Lowik CW, Kaijzel EL. In vivo optical approaches to angiogenesis imaging. *Angiogenesis* 2010; 13:135–47.

22. Dobrucki LW, de Muinck ED, Lndner JR, Sinusas AJ. Approaches to multimodality imaging of angiogenesis. *J Nucl Med* 2010; 51 Suppl 1:66S–79S.

23. Barrett T, Brechbiel M, Bernardo M, Choyke PL. MRI of tumor angiogenesis. *J Magn Reson Imaging* 2007; 26:235–49.

24. Daldrup-Link HE, Simon GH, Brasch RC. Imaging of tumor angiogenesis: current approaches and future prospects. *Curr Pharm Des* 2006; 12:2661–72.

25. Laking GR, Price PM. Positron emission tomographic imaging of angiogenesis and vascular function. *Br J Radiol* 2003; 76 Spec No 1:S50–9.

26. Van De Wiele C, Oltenfreiter R, De Winter O, Signore A, Siegers G, Dierckx RA. Tumor angiogenesis pathways: related clinical issues and implications for nuclear medicine imaging. *Eur J Nucl Med Mol Imaging* 2002; 29:699–709.

27. Lee TY, Purdie TG, Stewart E. CT imaging of angiogenesis. *Q J Nucl Med* 2003; 47:171–87.

28. Deshpande N, Pysz MA, Willmann JK. Molecular ultrasound assessment of tumor angiogenesis. *Angiogenesis* 2010; 13:175–88.

29. Eisenbrey JR, Forsberg F. Contrast-enhanced ultrasound for molecular imaging of angiogenesis. *Eur J Nucl Med Mol Imaging* 2010; Suppl 1:S138–46.

30. Liu Y, Yang Y, Zhang C. A concise review of magnetic resonance molecular imaging of tumor angiogenesis by targeting integrin avb3 with magnetic probes. *Int J Nanomedicien* 2013; 8:1083–93.

31. Danhier F, Le Breton A, Preat V. RGD-based strategies to target alpha(v) beta(3) integrin in cancer therapy and diagnosis. *Mol pharm* 2012; 9:2961–73.

32. Gaertner FC, Schwaiger M, Beer AJ. Molecular imaging of avb3 expression in cancer patients. *Q J Nucl Med Mol Imaging* 2010; 54:309–26.

33. Contois L, Akalu A, Brooks PC. Integrins as "functional hubs" in the regulation of pathological angiogenesis. *Semin Cancer Biol* 2009; 19:318–28.

34. Liu Z, Wang F. Development of RGD-based radiotracers for tumor imaging and therapy: translating from bench to bedside. *Curr Mol Med* 2013; 13:1487–1505.

35. Beer AJ, Schwaiger M. Imaging of integrin alphavbeta3 expression. *Cancer Metastasis Rev* 2008; 27:631–44.

Chapter

13

Reporter Genes

Amer M. Najjar, Laura J. Fromme, and Shahriar Yaghoubi

13.1 Introduction

Positron emission tomography (PET) is a noninvasive clinical imaging modality that can be combined with reporter gene expression to enable the specific and repetitive detection of a variety of cellular processes. These cellular processes include transcriptional regulation, signal transduction, protein-protein interactions, and cell trafficking and engraftment. The ability to detect these processes with PET reporter gene/probe systems also enables non-invasive monitoring of the pharmacokinetics and pharmacodynamics of therapeutics and their efficacy in vivo.

The concept of reporter gene imaging emerged from systems designed to image intrinsic enzymatic and metabolic processes and targets leading to the development of the reporter/radiotracer concept. The premise of reporter gene-based expression is based on the irreversible binding or entrapment and accumulation of reporter probes (radiotracers). These reporter probes are labeled with positron-emitting radionuclides. Accumulation of the probes in or at target cells is mediated by the catalytic activity of the reporter gene products (enzymes), their binding affinity to the reporter proteins or transport through reporter proteins. This reporter gene-mediated binding, accumulation, and retention of positron-emitting reporter probes in target cells enables repetitive spatial-temporal dynamic imaging of molecular and cellular events by PET.

Reporter-based imaging requires the transfer and expression of a reporter gene into target cells by transfection, electroporation, or transduction. These reporter genes are encoded within expression cassettes which initiate and control their expression. These control elements fall into two general categories: constitutive and conditional. Constitutively expressed reporters are used to "label" cells ex vivo for studies that require monitoring of trafficking and distribution patterns of the infused cells. The utility of this method has been most routinely illustrated in adoptive immunotherapy applications where T cells are labeled to determine their trafficking, biodistribution, and targeting patterns. It is also used in stem cell therapy applications to determine the long-term viability and therapeutic efficacy of infused stem cells.

Reporter gene expression driven by conditional tissue-specific promoters provides functional information about the target cells. Conditional promoters, for example, can provide information about the functional status of T cells related to their activation and proliferation and telomerase activity in tumor cells. PET reporters fall into three basic categories: enzyme-, receptor-, and transporter-based systems (Figure 13.1). Each system possesses advantages and limitations that have to be taken into account for any specific application. These factors must also be considered during image data analysis to ensure correct and objective interpretation of results.

13.2 Enzyme-Based Reporter Genes

Enzyme-based PET reporter systems are based on the conversion of radiolabeled substrates into impermeable polar molecules that consequently accumulate within the target cells that express the reporter gene. The continuous catalytic conversion of radiolabeled substrates by the enzymatic reporters results in focal intracellular accumulation that amplifies the PET signal and enhances the signal-to-noise ratio.

As a rule, the radiotracer must only be selectively catalyzed by the exogenously introduced enzymatic reporter and not by any other endogenous enzyme. Thus, endogenous enzymes must not catalyze the radiotracer molecules to prevent off-target or nonspecific accumulation of the substrates producing false "hot-spots."

Nucleotide kinases are the most extensively studied and applied group of PET reporter enzymes. Both mammalian and viral nucleotide kinases have been

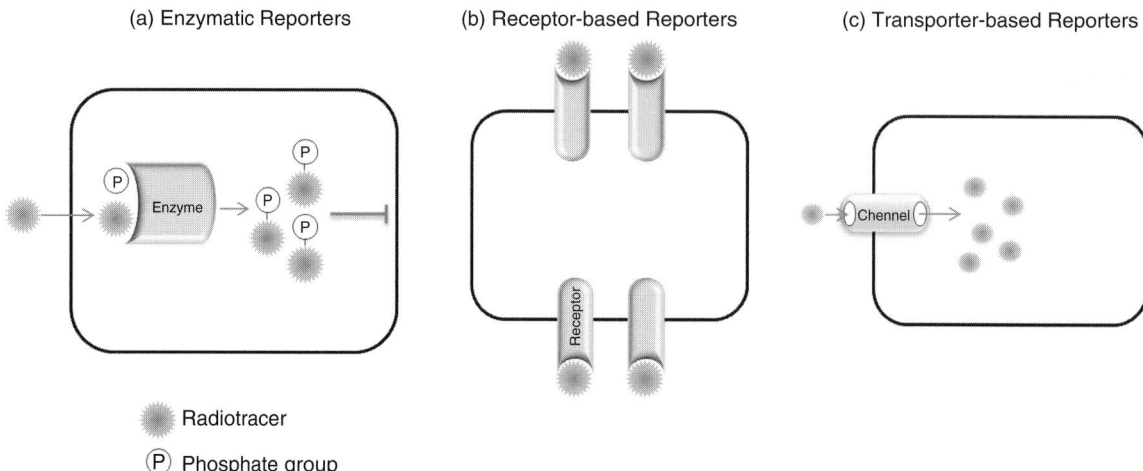

(a) Enzymatic Reporters **(b) Receptor-based Reporters** **(c) Transporter-based Reporters**

✳ Radiotracer

(P) Phosphate group

Figure 13.1 Three classes of PET reporters. (A) Enzymatic reporters are based on the conversion of radiotracers into impermeable molecules that accumulate specifically in target cells. (B) Receptor-based reporters systems are based on the specific binding of radiolabeled ligands to cell surface proteins. Radiotracer concentration is saturable being limited to the number of cell surface receptors. (C) Transporter-based reporter systems facilitate the active transport and intracellular accumulation of radioisotopes. Similar to enzyme-based receptors, transporters yield signal amplification as a consequence of exponential radiotracer accumulation.

adapted for use as reporter genes. Numerous variants of these enzymes have been produced by random and targeted mutagenesis to restrict or enhance their substrate specificity and catalytic activity. This has resulted in optimized sensitivity and specificity of detection by PET. Thymidine and cytidine kinases are the most well-established enzymatic reporters in experimental and clinical applications.

Thymidine kinase reporter genes are based on the selective and specific phosphorylation of pyrimidine and acycloguanosine nucleoside analogs to their monophosphate forms resulting in their entrapment and accumulation in target tissue expressing the enzyme (Figure 13.1A). This entrapment is facilitated by phosphorylation of the radiotracer and its enzymatic conversion into an impermeable polar product. Subsequent conversion of these monophosphorylated nucleosides into di- and tri-phosphates further enhances their intracellular entrapment. This focal accumulation of radioactivity can be detected noninvasively and repetitively in three dimensions using conventional preclinical and clinical PET instruments.

13.2.1 Herpes Simplex Virus 1 Thymidine Kinase

The feasibility of an enzyme-based PET reporter gene was first demonstrated with herpes simplex virus-1 thymidine kinase (HSV1tk). PET was utilized to report on the therapeutic and virus-mediated delivery of HSV1tk to target tissue using 5-iodo-2'-fluoro-2'deoxy-1-beta-D-arabino-furanosyl-uracil (FIAU) as the radiolabeled nucleoside probe. Subsequently, this approach was adapted to detect cell migration patterns and to report on tissue-specific gene expression by using the specific promoter-driven expression of HSV1tk in ex vivo modified cells expressing HSV1tk.

HSV1tk possesses a broad nucleoside substrate specificity which has been exploited to develop a wide range of radiolabeled probes (Table 13.1). These probes have been matched with variants of HSV1tk to maximize the catalytic rate of phosphorylation of the nucleoside substrates to enhance the rate of probe accumulation in target tissue. Wild-type HSV1tk exhibits maximal catalysis of pyrimidine analogs such as ^{124}I-FIAU and ^{18}F-FEAU. On the other hand, the sr39 variant of HSV1tk was selectively developed using random mutagenesis and selected for enhanced specificity toward the purine acycloguanosine derivatives. Thus, sr39tk exhibits maximal specificity for the acycloguanosine derivative probes ^{18}F-FHBG, ^{18}F-FACV, ^{18}F-FGCV, ^{18}F-FPCV, and ^{18}F-FHPG. Other variants of HSV1tk have been produced to exclusively restrict the specificity of the kinase toward acycloguanosine nucleotides. This refined specificity can potentially be utilized to

Table 13.1 Summary of Reporter/Probe Sets

Category	Reporter gene	Probe(s)	Mode of action	Reference
Enyzme	Wild-type HSV1tk	[18F]-FIAU	Nucleoside analog kinase	(18)
		[18F]-FACV		(27)
		[18F]-FGCV		(27)
		[18F]-FPCV		(28)
		[18F]-FHPG		(29,30)
		[18F]-FHBG		(25,61)
		[18F]-FMAU		
	sr39tk	[18F]-FHBG	Nucleoside analog kinase	(61)
	HSV1tk (A168H)	[18F]-FEAU	Nucleoside analog kinase	(31)
	dCK	[18F]-FEAU	Nucleoside analog kinase	(39)
		[18F]--FAC		(36)
		[18F]--FMAC		(36)
	hTK2	[18F]-FEAU	Nucleoside analog kinase	(34)
		[18F]-FIAU		(34)
		[18F]-FHBG		(34)
	hTK2 (N93D/L109F)	[18F]-FMAU	Nucleoside analog kinase	(35)
Receptor	Dopamine Receptor 2	[18F]-FESP	Cell surface receptor	(46)
	Somatostatin Receptor 2	[67Ga]/[68Ga]-octreotide		(42)
		[94mTc]-Demotate	Cell surface receptor	(43)
Transporter	NaI symporter (NIS)	Na[124I]	Transmembrane ion channel	(55)
	Norepinephrine transporter	[123I/124I]-MIBG	Neurotransmitter channel	(58,59)
		[11C]-hydroxyephidrine		(60)

Abbreviations:
[18F]-FIAU = 5-iodo-2'-[18F]fluoro-2'-deoxy-I-b-D-arabinofuranosyl-5-iodouracil
[18F]-FACV = 8-[18F]fluoroacyclovir
[18F]-FGCV = 8-[18F]fluoroganciclovir
[18F]-FPCV = 8-[18F]fluoro-9-[4-hydroxy-3-(hydroxymethy)-I-butyl]guanine
[18F]-FHPG = 9-[(3-[18F]fluoro-1-hydroxy-2-propoxy)methyl]guanine
[18F]-FHBG = 9-(4-[18F]fluoro-3-hydroxymethylbutyl)-guanine
[18F]-FMAU = 2'-deoxy-2'-[18F]-5-methyl-1-beta-L-arabinofuranosyluracil
[18F]-FEAU = [18F]-2'-fluoro-2'-deoxy-1-beta-D-beta-arabinofuranosyl-5-ethyluracil
[18F]-FESP = 3-(2'-[18F]fluoroethyl)spiperone
[18F]-FAC = 1-(2'-deoxy-2'-[18F]-fluoro-beta-L-arabinofuranosyl)cytosine
[18F]-FMAC = 1-(2'-deoxy-2'-[18F]-fluoro-beta-L-arabinofuranosyl)-5-methylcytosine
[123I/124I]-MIBG = [123I/124I]-metaiodobenzylguanidine
dCK = Deoxycytidine kinase
hTK2 (N93D/L109F) = human mitochondrial thymidine kinase type 2 mutant
hTK2 = human mitochondrial thymidine kinase type 2

image two independent events in the same subject by PET using HSV1tk variants with exclusive substrate specificities.

Unlike saturable receptor-based reporter genes, the enzymatic activity of HSV1tk yields constant and rapid substrate turnover leading to exponential signal amplification. This results in the entrapment and intracellular accumulation of the nucleoside radiotracers. Thus, the catalytic rate of phosphorylation is a major factor contributing to sensitivity of detection as determined by the signal-to-noise ratio.

A host immune response against HSV1-tk-expressing cells may limit the persistence or eradicate adoptively transferred cells in stem cell or immunotherapy applications, diminishing the efficacy of this therapeutic approach. This potential problem has prompted the development of non-immunogenic alternative reporter enzymes of human origin.

13.2.2 Mitochondrial Thymidine Kinase-2

Human thymidine kinase 2 (hTK2) is a mitochondrial enzyme that has been adapted for use as a PET reporter enzyme. It exhibits broader substrate specificity than the endogenous nuclear thymidine kinase 1 effectively catalyzing thymidine analogs such as FEAU and FIAU. Because of its human origin, hTK2 is potentially less immunogenic when utilized as a PET reporter and suitable for long-term repetitive clinical imaging. A cytoplasmic form of hTK2 (truncated N-terminal mitochondrial localization domain) can effectively phosphorylate FEAU and FIAU leading to their intracellular accumulation in target cells. However, the acycloguanosine nucleoside radiotracer FHBG is not readily catalyzed by hTK2. This suggests the reporter enzyme may potentially be used as a secondary reporter gene in conjunction with the sr39 or A168H variants of HSV1tk, which have inverse specificities for the acycloguanosine substrates.

The natural specificity of hTK2 for thymidine is a potential drawback to its application as a PET reporter. Its catalytic activity may upset homeostatic metabolism of intracellular thymidine and adversely affect replication-related cellular processes. To this end, a variant form of hTK2 containing a double mutation (N93D, L109F) has been specifically engineered to reduce the enzyme's specificity for the thymidine and deoxycytidine. This prevents altering endogenous nucleotide metabolism while maintaining its catalytic activity for FMAU. The restricted substrate specificity and probable nonimmunogenicity of this hTK2 variant promote its clinical application by prolonging the viability of target cells and enabling long-term longitudinal imaging.

13.2.3 Deoxycytidine Kinase

Deoxycytidine kinase (dCK) is a rate-limiting enzyme in the deoxyribonucleoside salvage pathway that produces and maintains intracellular levels of deoxyribonucleoside triphosphates (dNTPs) required for DNA synthesis. Its association with the cell cycle has made it an attractive drug target to inhibit cancer cell growth, and a number of nucleoside analogs (cytarabine, gemcitabine, decitabine, cladribine, and clofarabine) have been developed as drugs to inhibit cancer cell growth based on inhibition of dCK activity. Labeled forms of these drugs were subsequently developed to image human tumors that have elevated intrinsic deoxyribonucleoside salvage pathway activity. Cancer cells have been detected by PET using ^{18}F-labeled dCK substrate analogs such as 1-(2'-deoxy-2'-(18)F-fluoro-beta-L-arabinofuranosyl) cytosine ([^{18}F]-FAC) and 1-(2'-deoxy-2'-(18)F-fluoro-beta-L-arabinofuranosyl)-5-methylcytosine ([^{18}F]-FMAC) due to elevated dCK activity in these highly proliferating cells.

The availability of PET probes for imaging intrinsic dCK activity set the stage for utilizing this kinase as an enzymatic reporter gene. As dCK reporter gene probes, [^{18}F]-FAC and [^{18}F]-FMAC were selected based on their low susceptibility to deamination, specificity for recombinant dCK, high uptake in dCK-expressing cell lines, and biodistribution within intrinsic dCK-positive tissue.

Mutant forms of dCK have also been developed to shift catalytic activity toward pyrimidine nucleoside analogs. A triple mutant dCK (R104M, D133A, S74E) demonstrated newly established catalytic specificity for FEAU (equivalent to wild-type HSV1-tk), sensitivity to pyrimidine-based prodrugs (gemcitabine, Ara-C), and lack of specificity for the acycloguanosine substrates [^{18}F]-FHBG and ganciclovir. This enhanced catalytic activity was applied to image implanted hematopoietic stem cells for up to thirty-two weeks in a mouse model using L-FMAU without affecting the engraftment and differentiation potential of infused cells. Like hTK2, the human origin of dCK minimizes its immunogenic potential and enhances its potential application in long-term clinical PET imaging studies.

13.3 Receptor-Based Reporters

Receptor-based PET reporter genes rely on the binding of a positron-emitting probe to receptors expressed on the surface of target cells. Unlike intracellular enzymatic reporters, the radiolabeled probe is not required to cross the cellular membrane and is readily accessible to the cell surface receptor (Figure 13.1B). The mammalian somastatin receptor (SSTr) and the dopamine type 2 receptor (D2R) are the two most notably studied and applied PET receptor-based reporter genes. Their human origin and the availability of FDA-approved radiolabeled ligands enhance their potential clinical application.

13.3.1 Somastatin Receptor (SSTr)

Utilizing SSTr as a PET reporter is well-established. SSTr is a cell surface G-protein coupled receptor with widely distributed basal expression in a variety of tissues including brain, pancreas, kidney, spleen as well as neuroendocrine tumors. Activating SSTr induces signaling pathways that inhibit growth hormone release resulting in an antimitotic effect. Somatostatin, a 14-amino acid cyclic peptide, is the SSTr ligand. High levels of SSTr expression on human neuroendocrine tumors prompted the development of labeled somatostatin analogs for therapeutic and imaging purposes. Octreotide and Demotate are analogs derived from the original somatostatin sequence. They are composed of a minimized cyclic 4-amino acid receptor-binding sequence with an increased half-life in circulation and specificity for SSTr type 2A. Rapid radiolabeling techniques have been developed to produce [^{94m}Tc]-Demotate and [^{67}Ga]/[^{68}Ga]-Octreotide for PET imaging. The rapid renal clearance of the somatostatin analogs minimizes background activity compared to imaging agents that are slowly cleared via the heptobiliary route leading to long-lasting high background signal interference in the gastrointestinal tract.

13.3.2 Dopamine Type 2 Receptor (D2R)

The dopamine 2 receptor (D2R) is a G-protein coupled transmembrane protein ubiquitously expressed in the central nervous system. Given its central role in neurological disorders, radiolabeled ligands for PET imaging were developed as diagnostic agents for disorders such as schizophrenia. These probes, 3-(2-[^{18}F]fluoroethyl)spiperone (^{18}F-FESP) and ^{11}C-FLB 457, bind to D2R in extrastriatal regions of the brain.

The D2R ligand-receptor system has found application as a reporter gene system when expressed as a transgene in cells that do not naturally express the neuroreceptor. Virus-mediated transfer of D2R with HSV1tk encoded on separate vectors or together on bistronic vectors results in proportional uptake of [^{18}F]-FESP and [^{18}F]-FEAU, respectively. This dual reporter expression approach enables multitracer detection of reporter-expressing cells by PET.

Activation of D2R inhibits adenylyl cyclase resulting in the inhibition of cAMP formation. Therefore, expression of D2R as a PET reporter gene may potentially alter intracellular cAMP levels leading to the disruption of signaling pathways in transduced cells. This may introduce uncertainty in experimental outcome and in the interpretation of results as cellular behavior may be altered.

To circumvent this potential problem, a mutation has been introduced into the receptor, Asp80 to Ala (D2R80A), to eliminate its ability to stimulate downstream signaling pathways that modulate cAMP levels. D2R80A lacks downstream signaling activation capacity but maintains ligand binding affinity equivalent to the wild-type receptor. This feature enhances the utility of D2R as reporter gene by restricting its role solely to a radioligand receptor.

13.3.3 Other Receptor-Based Reporters

New forms of receptor-based reporter/probe systems have been described recently but have not yet been extensively evaluated or applied. One receptor-based PET reporter system is a chimeric protein composed of the carcinoembryonic antigen (CEA) fused to the cytoplasmic domains of the human transferrin receptor, CD5, or the human Fc gamma RIIb receptor. This receptor is internalized upon binding of radiolabeled anti-CEA antibody. PET imaging with ^{124}I- or ^{64}Cu-single chain Fv-Fc antibody fragment was demonstrated in vivo in mice bearing tumor xenografts.

The human estrogen receptor (hER) has also been evaluated as a receptor-based reporter gene in conjunction with ^{18}F-labeled estradiol (FES). The DNA-binding domain of the human estrogen receptor is truncated leaving only the ligand (hERL)-binding region which lacks any functional activity as a transcription factor.

Another receptor imaging system is based on cell surface expression of antibody fragments that can irreversibly bind to radiolabeled chelators – 1,4,7,10-tetraazacyclodocecane-N,N',N'',N'''-tetraacetic acid (DOTA) antibody reporter 1 (DAbR1). This receptor is composed of a single-chain Fv (scFv) fragment of the anti-Y-DOTA antibody anchored on the cell surface with the human T cell CD4 transmembrane domain. The reporter probe, yttrium-(S)-2-(4-acrylamidobenzyl)-DOTA, binds irreversibly to the receptor via a cysteine residue in the scFv region of the antibody receptor.

13.4 Transporter-Based Reporters

Similar to enzyme-based reporters, transporter-based reporter genes have the advantage of signal amplification by facilitating accumulative influx and intracellular concentration of radiotracers (Figure 13.1C). In addition, transporters provide the advantage of being readily accessible on the cell surface circumventing the requirement for transmembrane transport of the radiotracer before catalysis by cytoplasmic reporter enzymes. Two human transmembrane transporters have been utilized as PET reporters – the sodium iodide symporter (NIS) and the norepinephrine transporter (NET).

13.4.1 Sodium Iodide Symporter (NIS)

NIS is an 87 kDa transmembrane glycoprotein with 13 transmembrane domains that transport sodium and iodide ions at a 2:1 ratio. NIS is endogenously expressed in various tissues including the thyroid, stomach, kidney epithelium, and salivary gland. The intrinsic ability of the thyroid gland to take up iodide opened the way for the development of diagnostic and targeted therapeutic applications based on intracellular transport of radioactive iodide (^{123}I-, ^{124}I-, and ^{131}I-) and other anions ($^{88m}TcO_4^-$). This approach led to the cross utilization of NIS as a PET reporter gene expressed in exogenously transduced tissues. Na^{124}I has been routinely used to image cells transduced with the NIS gene. Numerous applications of NIS-based reporter gene include monitoring of adenoviral gene transfer to the heart, telomerase activity in tumor cells, stem cell persistence and engraftment, and macrophage migration in an animal model of inflammation.

13.4.2 Norepinephrine Transporter (NET)

NET is a transmembrane transporter that facilitates the intracellular transfer of norepinephrine, dopamine, and epinephrine at presynaptic terminals to terminate neurotransmitter-mediated signaling. The exclusive expression of NET within the central and peripheral sympathetic nervous system has led to successful clinical imaging with radiolabeled neurotransmitter analogs such as $^{123/124}$I-metaiodobenzylguanidine (MIBG) and ^{11}C-hydroxyephidrine with high signal-to-background. This clinical imaging methodology has facilitated the application of NET as a PET reporter gene.

13.5 Criteria for Effective Reporter Gene Imaging

Effective reporter gene imaging is dependent on radiotracer volume of distribution. Focal accumulation of radiotracer at target sites (where reporter genes are expressed) and rapid clearance of radiotracer from nontarget tissue determine the signal-to-noise ratio and, thus, the sensitivity and specificity of detection.

Several factors have to be taken into consideration in reporter gene imaging applications.

1. In enzyme- and transporter-based systems, radiotracers must be exclusively and specifically catalyzed or transported by the reporter (as measured by k_{cat}/K_m). Receptor-based systems must exhibit specific and high binding affinity ($1/K_d$) to the radioligand. This aspect reduces off-target and nonspecific accumulation of probe to minimize background radiotracer levels (ideally $K_1 = k_2$ in a single compartment model of probe distribution). This scenario yields a favorable volume of distribution that maximizes the signal-to-noise ratio at target sites (where $K_1 \gg k_2$) and translates into enhanced signal contrast (sensitivity) and increased certainty (specificity) in identifying positive events.

2. The reporter gene product must be highly specific and restricted to interacting only with the probe. Reporter gene products must not interfere with intrinsic metabolic pathways by catalyzing, binding, or transporting endogenous molecules. Such interactions may adversely interfere with intrinsic cellular processes that regulate replication, differentiation, or metabolism, thereby introducing uncertainty in experimental outcome.

3. The level of reporter gene expression, catalytic activity of enzymatic reporters, and receptor density are important determinants of sensitivity. Enzyme- and transporter-based systems yield exponential amplification of signal due to constant turnover and intracellular accumulation of radiotracer molecules. In contrast, receptor-based reporter gene imaging is dependent on binding potential (BP), which is a combined measure of available receptor density and the affinity of the radioligand to that receptor. Thus, PET signal intensity is proportional to receptor density and approaches a saturation limit based on the number of available receptors.

Reporter genes provide crucial information about spatial and temporal dynamics of cellular processes through noninvasive and repetitive PET imaging. Minimizing uncertainty in result interpretation is critical and highly dependent on sensitivity and specificity of detection.

Further Reading

1. Ponomarev, V., Doubrovin, M., Lyddane, C., Beresten, T., Balatoni, J., Bornman, W., Finn, R., Akhurst, T., Larson, S., Blasberg, R., Sadelain, M., and Tjuvajev, J. G. (2001) Imaging TCR-dependent NFAT-mediated T-cell activation with positron emission tomography in vivo. *Neoplasia* 3, 480–488.

2. Holland, J. P., Cumming, P., and Vasdev, N. (2012) PET of signal transduction pathways in cancer. *J Nucl Med* 53, 1333–1336.

3. Massoud, T. F., Paulmurugan, R., and Gambhir, S. S. (2010) A molecularly engineered split reporter for imaging protein-protein interactions with positron emission tomography. *Nat Med* 16, 921–926.

4. Dotti, G., Tian, M., Savoldo, B., Najjar, A., Cooper, L. J., Jackson, J., Smith, A., Mawlawi, O., Uthamanthil, R., Borne, A., Brammer, D., Paolillo, V., Alauddin, M., Gonzalez, C., Steiner, D., Decker, W. K., Marini, F., Kornblau, S., Bollard, C. M., Shpall, E. J., and Gelovani, J. G. (2009) Repetitive noninvasive monitoring of HSV1-tk-expressing T cells intravenously infused into nonhuman primates using positron emission tomography and computed tomography with 18F-FEAU. *Mol Imaging* 8, 230–237.

5. McCracken, M. N., Gschweng, E. H., Nair-Gill, E., McLaughlin, J., Cooper, A. R., Riedinger, M., Cheng, D., Nosala, C., Kohn, D. B., and Witte, O. N. (2013) Long-term in vivo monitoring of mouse and human hematopoietic stem cell engraftment with a human positron emission tomography reporter gene. *Proc Natl Acad Sci USA* 110, 1857–1862.

6. Wang, F., Wang, Z., Hida, N., Kiesewetter, D. O., Ma, Y., Yang, K., Rong, P., Liang, J., Tian, J., Niu, G., and Chen, X. (2014) A cyclic HSV1-TK reporter for real-time PET imaging of apoptosis. *Proc Natl Acad Sci USA* 111, 5165–5170.

7. Gambhir, S. S. (2002) Molecular imaging of cancer with positron emission tomography. *Nat Rev Cancer* 2, 683–693.

8. Gelovani Tjuvajev, J., and Blasberg, R. G. (2003) In vivo imaging of molecular-genetic targets for cancer therapy. *Cancer Cell* 3, 327–332.

9. Dobrenkov, K., Olszewska, M., Likar, Y., Shenker, L., Gunset, G., Cai, S., Pillarsetty, N., Hricak, H., Sadelain, M., and Ponomarev, V. (2008) Monitoring the efficacy of adoptively transferred prostate cancer-targeted human T lymphocytes with PET and bioluminescence imaging. *J Nucl Med* 49, 1162–1170

10. Yaghoubi, S. S., Jensen, M. C., Satyamurthy, N., Budhiraja, S., Paik, D., Czernin, J., and Gambhir, S. S. (2009) Noninvasive detection of therapeutic cytolytic T cells with 18F-FHBG PET in a patient with glioma. *Nat Clin Pract Oncol* 6, 53–58.

11. Koehne, G., Doubrovin, M., Doubrovina, E., Zanzonico, P., Gallardo, H. F., Ivanova, A., Balatoni, J., Teruya-Feldstein, J., Heller, G., May, C., Ponomarev, V., Ruan, S., Finn, R., Blasberg, R. G., Bornmann, W., Riviere, I., Sadelain, M., O'Reilly, R. J., Larson, S. M., and Tjuvajev, J. G. (2003) Serial in vivo imaging of the targeted migration of human HSV-TK-transduced antigen-specific lymphocytes. *Nat Biotechnol* 21, 405–413.

12. Perin, E. C., Tian, M., Marini, F. C., III, Silva, G. V., Zheng, Y., Baimbridge, F., Quan, X., Fernandes, M. R., Gahremanpour, A., Young, D., Paolillo, V., Mukhopadhyay, U., Borne, A. T., Uthamanthil, R., Brammer, D., Jackson, J., Decker, W. K., Najjar, A. M., Thomas, M. W., Volgin, A., Rabinovich, B., Soghomonyan, S., Jeong, H. J., Rios, J. M., Steiner, D., Robinson, S., Mawlawi, O., Pan, T., Stafford, J., Kundra, V., Li, C., Alauddin, M. M., Willerson, J. T., Shpall, E., and Gelovani, J. G. (2011) Imaging long-term fate of intramyocardially implanted mesenchymal stem cells in a porcine myocardial infarction model. *PLoS One* 6, e22949.

13. Sun, N., Lee, A., and Wu, J. C. (2009) Long term non-invasive imaging of embryonic stem cells using reporter genes. *Nat Protoc* 4, 1192–1201.

14. Gyongyosi, M., Blanco, J., Marian, T., Tron, L., Petnehazy, O., Petrasi, Z., Hemetsberger, R., Rodriguez, J., Font, G., Pavo, I. J., Kertesz, I., Balkay, L., Pavo, N., Posa, A., Emri, M., Galuska, L., Kraitchman, D. L., Wojta, J., Huber, K., and Glogar, D. (2008) Serial noninvasive in vivo positron emission tomographic tracking of percutaneously intramyocardially injected autologous porcine mesenchymal stem cells modified for transgene reporter gene expression. *Circ Cardiovasc Imaging* 1, 94–103.

15. Templin, C., Zweigerdt, R., Schwanke, K., Olmer, R., Ghadri, J. R., Emmert, M. Y., Muller, E., Kuest, S. M., Cohrs, S., Schibli, R., Kronen, P., Hilbe, M., Reinisch, A., Strunk, D., Haverich, A., Hoerstrup, S., Luscher, T. F., Kaufmann, P. A., Landmesser, U., and Martin, U. (2012) Transplantation and tracking of human-induced pluripotent stem cells in a pig model of myocardial infarction: assessment of cell survival, engraftment, and distribution by hybrid single photon emission computed tomography/computed tomography of sodium iodide symporter transgene expression. *Circulation* 126, 430–439.

16. Groot-Wassink, T., Aboagye, E. O., Wang, Y., Lemoine, N. R., Keith, W. N., and Vassaux, G. (2004) Noninvasive imaging of the transcriptional activities of human telomerase promoter fragments in mice. *Cancer Res* 64, 4906–4911.

17. Riesco-Eizaguirre, G., De la Vieja, A., Rodriguez, I., Miranda, S., Martin-Duque, P., Vassaux, G., and Santisteban, P. (2011) Telomerase-driven expression

of the sodium iodide symporter (NIS) for in vivo radioiodide treatment of cancer: a new broad-spectrum NIS-mediated antitumor approach. *J Clin Endocrinol Metab* 96, E1435–1443.

18. Tjuvajev, J. G., Avril, N., Oku, T., Sasajima, T., Miyagawa, T., Joshi, R., Safer, M., Beattie, B., DiResta, G., Daghighian, F., Augensen, F., Koutcher, J., Zweit, J., Humm, J., Larson, S. M., Finn, R., and Blasberg, R. (1998) Imaging herpes virus thymidine kinase gene transfer and expression by positron emission tomography. *Cancer Res* 58, 4333–4341.

19. Penuelas, I., Haberkorn, U., Yaghoubi, S., and Gambhir, S. S. (2005) Gene therapy imaging in patients for oncological applications. *Eur J Nucl Med Mol Imaging* 32 Suppl 2, S384–403.

20. Jacobs, A., Voges, J., Reszka, R., Lercher, M., Gossmann, A., Kracht, L., Kaestle, C., Wagner, R., Wienhard, K., and Heiss, W. D. (2001) Positron-emission tomography of vector-mediated gene expression in gene therapy for gliomas. *Lancet* 358, 727–729.

21. Tjuvajev, J. G., Finn, R., Watanabe, K., Joshi, R., Oku, T., Kennedy, J., Beattie, B., Koutcher, J., Larson, S., and Blasberg, R. G. (1996) Noninvasive imaging of herpes virus thymidine kinase gene transfer and expression: a potential method for monitoring clinical gene therapy. *Cancer Res* 56, 4087–4095.

22. Sun, X., Annala, A. J., Yaghoubi, S. S., Barrio, J. R., Nguyen, K. N., Toyokuni, T., Satyamurthy, N., Namavari, M., Phelps, M. E., Herschman, H. R., and Gambhir, S. S. (2001) Quantitative imaging of gene induction in living animals. *Gene Ther* 8, 1572–1579.

23. Serganova, I., Doubrovin, M., Vider, J., Ponomarev, V., Soghomonyan, S., Beresten, T., Ageyeva, L., Serganov, A., Cai, S., Balatoni, J., Blasberg, R., and Gelovani, J. (2004) Molecular imaging of temporal dynamics and spatial heterogeneity of hypoxia-inducible factor-1 signal transduction activity in tumors in living mice. *Cancer Res* 64, 6101–6108.

24. Soghomonyan, S., Hajitou, A., Rangel, R., Trepel, M., Pasqualini, R., Arap, W., Gelovani, J. G., and Alauddin, M. M. (2007) Molecular PET imaging of HSV1-tk reporter gene expression using [18F]FEAU. *Nat Protoc* 2, 416–423.

25. Alauddin, M. M., and Conti, P. S. (1998) Synthesis and preliminary evaluation of 9-(4-[18F]-fluoro-3-hydroxymethylbutyl)guanine ([18F]FHBG): a new potential imaging agent for viral infection and gene therapy using PET. *Nucl Med Biol* 25, 175–180.

26. Yaghoubi, S., Barrio, J. R., Dahlbom, M., Iyer, M., Namavari, M., Satyamurthy, N., Goldman, R., Herschman, H. R., Phelps, M. E., and Gambhir, S. S. (2001) Human pharmacokinetic and dosimetry studies of [(18)F]FHBG: a reporter probe for imaging herpes simplex virus type-1 thymidine kinase reporter gene expression. *J Nucl Med* 42, 1225–1234.

27. Gambhir, S. S., Barrio, J. R., Wu, L., Iyer, M., Namavari, M., Satyamurthy, N., Bauer, E., Parrish, C., MacLaren, D. C., Borghei, A. R., Green, L. A., Sharfstein, S., Berk, A. J., Cherry, S. R., Phelps, M. E., and Herschman, H. R. (1998) Imaging of adenoviral-directed herpes simplex virus type 1 thymidine kinase reporter gene expression in mice with radiolabeled ganciclovir. *J Nucl Med* 39, 2003–2011.

28. Kang, K. W., Min, J. J., Chen, X., and Gambhir, S. S. (2005) Comparison of [14C]FMAU, [3H]FEAU, [14C]FIAU, and [3H]PCV for monitoring reporter gene expression of wild type and mutant herpes simplex virus type 1 thymidine kinase in cell culture. *Mol Imaging Biol* 7, 296–303.

29. Alauddin, M. M., Conti, P. S., Mazza, S. M., Hamzeh, F. M., and Lever, J. R. (1996) 9-[(3-[18F]-fluoro-1-hydroxy-2-propoxy)methyl]guanine ([18F]-FHPG): a potential imaging agent of viral infection and gene therapy using PET. *Nucl Med Biol* 23, 787–792.

30. Alauddin, M. M., Shahinian, A., Kundu, R. K., Gordon, E. M., and Conti, P. S. (1999) Evaluation of 9-[(3-18F-fluoro-1-hydroxy-2-propoxy)methyl]guanine ([18F]-FHPG) in vitro and in vivo as a probe for PET imaging of gene incorporation and expression in tumors. *Nucl Med Biol* 26, 371–376.

31. Najjar, A. M., Nishii, R., Maxwell, D. S., Volgin, A., Mukhopadhyay, U., Bornmann, W. G., Tong, W., Alauddin, M., and Gelovani, J. G. (2009) Molecular-genetic PET imaging using an HSV1-tk mutant reporter gene with enhanced specificity to acycloguanosine nucleoside analogs. *J Nucl Med* 50, 409–416.

32. Traversari, C., Marktel, S., Magnani, Z., Mangia, P., Russo, V., Ciceri, F., Bonini, C., and Bordignon, C. (2007) The potential immunogenicity of the TK suicide gene does not prevent full clinical benefit associated with the use of TK-transduced donor lymphocytes in HSCT for hematologic malignancies. *Blood* 109, 4708–4715.

33. Berger, C., Flowers, M. E., Warren, E. H., and Riddell, S. R. (2006) Analysis of transgene-specific immune responses that limit the in vivo persistence of adoptively transferred HSV-TK-modified donor T cells after allogeneic hematopoietic cell transplantation. *Blood* 107, 2294–2302.

34. Ponomarev, V., Doubrovin, M., Shavrin, A., Serganova, I., Beresten, T., Ageyeva, L., Cai, C., Balatoni, J., Alauddin, M., and Gelovani, J. (2007) A human-derived reporter gene for noninvasive imaging in humans: mitochondrial thymidine kinase type 2. *J Nucl Med* 48, 819–826.

35. Campbell, D. O., Yaghoubi, S. S., Su, Y., Lee, J. T., Auerbach, M. S., Herschman, H., Satyamurthy, N., Czernin, J., Lavie, A., and Radu, C. G. (2012) Structure-guided engineering of human thymidine kinase 2 as a positron emission tomography reporter gene for enhanced phosphorylation of non-natural thymidine analog reporter probe. *J Biol Chem* 287, 446–454.

36. Schwarzenberg, J., Radu, C. G., Benz, M., Fueger, B., Tran, A. Q., Phelps, M. E., Witte, O. N., Satyamurthy, N., Czernin, J., and Schiepers, C. (2011) Human biodistribution and radiation dosimetry of novel PET probes targeting the deoxyribonucleoside salvage pathway. *Eur J Nucl Med Mol Imaging* 38, 711–721.

37. Leung, K. (2004) 1-(2'-Deoxy-2'-[18F]fluoroarabinofuranosyl)cytosine. Molecular Imaging and Contrast Agent Database (MICAD). National Center for Biotechnology Information, Bethesda, MD.

38. Shu, C. J., Campbell, D. O., Lee, J. T., Tran, A. Q., Wengrod, J. C., Witte, O. N., Phelps, M. E., Satyamurthy, N., Czernin, J., and Radu, C. G. (2010) Novel PET probes specific for deoxycytidine kinase. *J Nucl Med* 51, 1092–1098.

39. Likar, Y., Zurita, J., Dobrenkov, K., Shenker, L., Cai, S., Neschadim, A., Medin, J. A., Sadelain, M., Hricak, H., and Ponomarev, V. (2010) A new pyrimidine-specific reporter gene: a mutated human deoxycytidine kinase suitable for PET during treatment with acycloguanosine-based cytotoxic drugs. *J Nucl Med* 51, 1395–1403.

40. Iyidogan, P., and Lutz, S. (2008) Systematic exploration of active site mutations on human deoxycytidine kinase substrate specificity. *Biochemistry* 47, 4711–4720.

41. Yamada, Y., Post, S. R., Wang, K., Tager, H. S., Bell, G. I., and Seino, S. (1992) Cloning and functional characterization of a family of human and mouse somatostatin receptors expressed in brain, gastrointestinal tract, and kidney. *Proc Natl Acad Sci USA* 89, 251–255.

42. Stolz, B., Smith-Jones, P. M., Albert, R., Reist, H., Macke, H., and Bruns, C. (1994) Biological characterisation of [67Ga] or [68Ga] labelled DFO-octreotide (SDZ 216–927) for PET studies of somatostatin receptor positive tumors. *Hormone and metabolic research = Hormon-und Stoffwechselforschung = Hormones et metabolisme* 26, 453–459.

43. Rogers, B. E., Parry, J. J., Andrews, R., Cordopatis, P., Nock, B. A., and Maina, T. (2005) MicroPET imaging of gene transfer with a somatostatin receptor-based reporter gene and (94m)Tc-Demotate 1. *J Nucl Med* 46, 1889–1897.

44. Wienhard, K., Coenen, H. H., Pawlik, G., Rudolf, J., Laufer, P., Jovkar, S., Stocklin, G., and Heiss, W. D. (1990) PET studies of dopamine receptor distribution using [18F]fluoroethylspiperone: findings in disorders related to the dopaminergic system. *Journal of Neural Transmission. General Section* 81, 195–213.

45. Halldin, C., Farde, L., Hogberg, T., Mohell, N., Hall, H., Suhara, T., Karlsson, P., Nakashima, Y., and Swahn, C. G. (1995) Carbon-11-FLB 457: a radioligand for extrastriatal D2 dopamine receptors. *J Nucl Med* 36, 1275–1281.

46. MacLaren, D. C., Gambhir, S. S., Satyamurthy, N., Barrio, J. R., Sharfstein, S., Toyokuni, T., Wu, L., Berk, A. J., Cherry, S. R., Phelps, M. E., and Herschman, H. R. (1999) Repetitive, non-invasive imaging of the dopamine D2 receptor as a reporter gene in living animals. *Gene Ther* 6, 785–91.

47. Liang, Q., Gotts, J., Satyamurthy, N., Barrio, J., Phelps, M. E., Gambhir, S. S., and Herschman, H. R. (2002) Noninvasive, repetitive, quantitative measurement of gene expression from a bicistronic message by positron emission tomography, following gene transfer with adenovirus. *Mol Ther* 6, 73–82.

48. Liang, Q., Satyamurthy, N., Barrio, J. R., Toyokuni, T., Phelps, M. P., Gambhir, S. S., and Herschman, H. R. (2001) Noninvasive, quantitative imaging in living animals of a mutant dopamine D2 receptor reporter gene in which ligand binding is uncoupled from signal transduction. *Gene Ther* 8, 1490–1498.

49. Kummer, C., Winkeler, A., Dittmar, C., Bauer, B., Rueger, M. A., Rueckriem, B., Heneka, M. T., Vollmar, S., Wienhard, K., Fraefel, C., Heiss, W. D., and Jacobs, A. H. (2007) Multitracer positron emission tomographic imaging of exogenous gene expression mediated by a universal herpes simplex virus 1 amplicon vector. *Mol Imaging* 6, 181–192.

50. Barat, B., Kenanova, V. E., Olafsen, T., and Wu, A. M. (2011) Evaluation of two internalizing carcinoembryonic antigen reporter genes for molecular imaging. *Mol Imaging Biol* 13, 526–535.

51. Kenanova, V., Barat, B., Olafsen, T., Chatziioannou, A., Herschman, H. R., Braun, J., and Wu, A. M. (2009) Recombinant carcinoembryonic antigen as a reporter gene for molecular imaging. *Eur J Nucl Med Mol Imaging* 36, 104–114.

52. Furukawa, T., Lohith, T. G., Takamatsu, S., Mori, T., Tanaka, T., and Fujibayashi, Y. (2006) Potential of the FES-hERL PET reporter gene system – basic evaluation for gene therapy monitoring. *Nucl Med Biol* 33, 145–151.

53. Lohith, T. G., Furukawa, T., Mori, T., Kobayashi, M., and Fujibayashi, Y. (2008) Basic evaluation of FES-hERL PET tracer-reporter gene system for in vivo monitoring of adenoviral-mediated gene therapy. *Mol Imaging Biol* 10, 245–252.

54. Wei, L. H., Olafsen, T., Radu, C., Hildebrandt, I. J., McCoy, M. R., Phelps, M. E., Meares, C., Wu, A. M.,

63

Czernin, J., and Weber, W. A. (2008) Engineered antibody fragments with infinite affinity as reporter genes for PET imaging. *J Nucl Med* 49, 1828–1835.

55. Groot-Wassink, T., Aboagye, E. O., Wang, Y., Lemoine, N. R., Reader, A. J., and Vassaux, G. (2004) Quantitative imaging of Na/I symporter transgene expression using positron emission tomography in the living animal. *Mol Ther* 9, 436–442.

56. Rao, V. P., Miyagi, N., Ricci, D., Carlson, S. K., Morris, J. C., 3rd, Federspiel, M. J., Bailey, K. R., Russell, S. J., and McGregor, C. G. (2007) Sodium iodide symporter (hNIS) permits molecular imaging of gene transduction in cardiac transplantation. *Transplantation* 84, 1662–1666.

57. Lee, H. W., Jeon, Y. H., Hwang, M. H., Kim, J. E., Park, T. I., Ha, J. H., Lee, S. W., Ahn, B. C., and Lee, J. (2013) Dual reporter gene imaging for tracking macrophage migration using the human sodium iodide symporter and an enhanced firefly luciferase in a murine inflammation model. *Mol Imaging Biol* 15, 703–712.

58. Doubrovin, M. M., Doubrovina, E. S., Zanzonico, P., Sadelain, M., Larson, S. M., and O'Reilly, R. J.

(2007) In vivo imaging and quantitation of adoptively transferred human antigen-specific T cells transduced to express a human norepinephrine transporter gene. *Cancer Res* 67, 11959–11969.

59. Brader, P., Kelly, K. J., Chen, N., Yu, Y. A., Zhang, Q., Zanzonico, P., Burnazi, E. M., Ghani, R. E., Serganova, I., Hricak, H., Szalay, A. A., Fong, Y., and Blasberg, R. G. (2009) Imaging a genetically engineered oncolytic vaccinia virus (GLV-1h99) using a human norepinephrine transporter reporter gene. *Clin Cancer Res* 15, 3791–3801.

60. Buursma, A. R., Beerens, A. M., de Vries, E. F., van Waarde, A., Rots, M. G., Hospers, G. A., Vaalburg, W., and Haisma, H. J. (2005) The human norepinephrine transporter in combination with 11C-m-hydroxyephedrine as a reporter gene/reporter probe for PET of gene therapy. *J Nucl Med* 46, 2068–2075.

61. Yaghoubi, S. S., and Gambhir, S. S. (2006) PET imaging of herpes simplex virus type 1 thymidine kinase (HSV1-tk) or mutant HSV1-sr39tk reporter gene expression in mice and humans using [18F]FHBG. *Nat Protoc* 1, 3069–3075.

Chapter 14

Stem Cell Tracking

Daniel Golovko, Ramsha Khan, and Heike Daldrup-Link

Stem cell therapies aim to replace abnormal, injured, or lost cells in organs with little or no capacity for self-renewal and provide hope for cures of devastating diseases with previously presumed irreversible functional loss, such as myocardial or brain infarction, blindness, paraplegia, diabetes mellitus, and degenerative or post-traumatic bone/ cartilage defects, among many others. In order to treat a cellular and/or functional deficit in a selected target organ, stem cells or stem-cell-derived cell populations are administered systemically (e.g. into the blood system), into a cavity (e.g. into a brain ventricle), or directly into target tissue (e.g. into myocardium). Many questions arise about the fate of the administered cells. Do the stem cells actually end up where they are desired (homing)? Do they survive? Do they integrate themselves with the host tissue (engraftment)? If undifferentiated stem cells are transplanted, do these cells differentiate into the desired specialized progenies and restore the impaired function of the target tissue? Does the host's immune system tolerate or reject the transplanted cells? Noninvasive imaging techniques can address these questions and help to develop and monitor successful approaches for stem-cell-mediated tissue regeneration.

14.1 Methods to Visualize Stem Cell Homing and Engraftment

There are various classical methods of showing distribution of stem cells in the body. Most rely on introducing a marker into the graft material that can be specifically stained after explantation. One common method is the transfection of stem cells with a plasmid containing *lacZ*. *lacZ* encodes β-galactosidase, an enzyme not normally found in human cells. After explantation, fixation, and staining of material to be examined, marked cells will stain while unmarked cells will not. This method is applicable only in animal models. Another common pre-clinical method

is the transfection of stem cells with luciferase genes. Luciferase catalyzes a two-step chemical reaction of the substrate luciferin, which leads to bioluminescence detectable in vivo by an optical imaging system. Photon generation following intravenous administration of luciferin takes place exclusively at the site of luciferase expression; therefore, the target-to-background signal ratio is extremely high. Bioluminescence imaging has been used for cell tracking in small animal models. However, limitations for human application for cell tracking are poor spatial resolution, the need to inject high doses of luciferin to generate a contrast effect, and potential immunogenicity of the foreign gene protein, luciferase.

Strategies to overcome these limitations for translational and clinical applications are :

1. Ex vivo labeling of the stem cells with a contrast agent or radiotracer prior to implantation;
2. Utilizing a transporter uniquely located on the stem cell to mediate contrast agent or radiotracer uptake after systemic injection; and
3. Genetically varying the stem cell to express a substrate that is primarily active as a contrast agent or that traps or activates a contrast agent or radiotracer.

14.1.1 Ex Vivo Labeling of the Stem Cells with a Contrast Agent or Radiotracer Prior to Implantation

Homing and engraftment of stem cells has been predominately monitored through labeling cells prior to implantation. Although standard radiotracers provide very high sensitivity and specificity, rapid radioactivity decay limits applications in this context because cell tracking can only be visualized for hours or a few days after transplantation. Stem cells can also be labeled with clinically applicable fluorescent agents, such as indocyanine green, to allow in vivo tracking with optical imaging. However, the limited tissue penetration of most fluorescent labels limits potential clinical applications to specific body parts (e.g. hands, breast tissue) and/or endoscopy-based or intraoperative approaches.

Photoacoustic imaging approaches may overcome some of these limitations. In photoacoustic imaging, nonionizing laser light pulses are sent into biological tissues. The delivered energy is converted to heat, leading to ultrasound emission, which can be detected by ultrasound transducers to form an image ("light in – ultrasound out"). Photoacoustic imaging may provide better tissue penetration and anatomic information than optical imaging alone. Photoacoustic imaging of nanorod-labeled mesenchymal stem cells has been recently reported in mouse models.

Most direct stem cell labeling and tracking approaches have been performed with contrast agents for MR imaging. MR contrast agents have either a predominant T_1 effect or a predominant T_2 effect. Most investigators prefer T_2 contrast agents for cell labeling, such as superparamagnetic particles of iron oxides (SPIO), because they provide substantially higher sensitivity for cell detection compared to standard Gd-chelates. When introduced into tissue, SPIO produce local magnetic field inhomogeneities which disrupt the local magnetic field. Consequently, the T_2^* and T_2 relaxation times are primarily reduced in the respective anatomical area which leads to hypointense MR signal (decrease in signal intensity, darker color in the image) on T_2^* and T_2-weighted MR images. There have been numerous applications of MR-based tracking of SPIO-labeled stem cells in both the pre-clinical and clinical settings. The major advantage of this technique is that stem cells can be tracked for many days to weeks (Figure 14.1). An important drawback is that the signal of the contrast agent label does not change when the stem cells undergo an apoptosis, that is one cannot distinguish between viable or dead stem cells. In addition, magnetic field inhomogeneities due to metallic implants or hemosiderin deposits after hemorrhage cannot be differentiated from SPIO contrast on T_2-weighted MR images and may cause false positive findings.

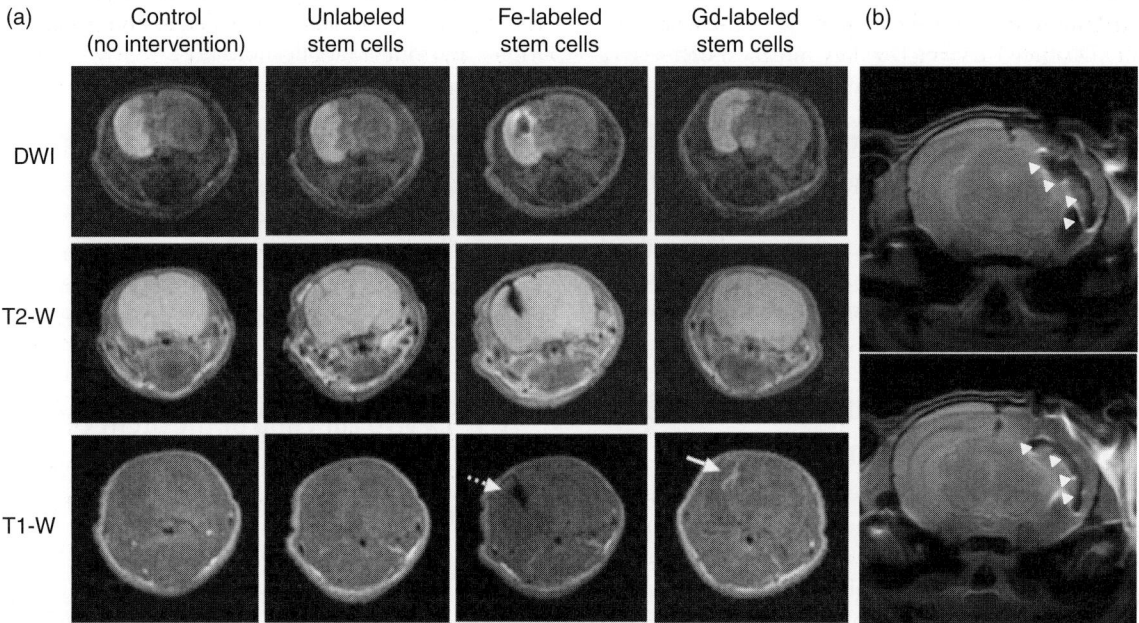

Figure 14.1 (A) Coronal diffusion weighted (DWI), T2-weighted (T2-W) and T1-weighted (T1-W) MR images of a right middle cerebral artery (MCA) stroke in a mouse after direct injection of 100,000 unlabeled, iron oxide nanoparticle (Fe) labeled and Gd-labeled stem cells into the infarct area. Iron oxide nanoparticle-labeled stem cells (dashed arrow) provide a negative (dark) signal effect, which exceeds the volume of the transplanted cells, a so-called blooming effect. Gd-labeled cells (white arrow) can be delineated more accurately and cannot be confused with local hemorrhage or accidental air injection. However, detection of the Gd-labeled cells is more difficult compared to detection of Fe-labeled cells due to lower sensitivity of the MRI technique to detect Gd-labeled cells. (B) High resolution T2-weighted MR scan (in plane resolution 100 μm) of the brain of another mouse after stereotactic injection of 200,000 iron oxide nanoparticle labeled stem cells into the left brain hemisphere (arrowheads).

Stem cells can also be labeled with standard T_1 contrast agents, typically gadolinium (Gd) chelates that, upon interaction with protons, shorten T_1 relaxation times. A shorter T_1 time leads to spins recovering faster which leads to higher (brighter) signal on T_1-weighted MR images. Gd-based contrast agents have been applied for a large variety of stem cell tracking applications. One advantage is the positive signal of the labeled cells with fewer false positive findings compared to SPIO. However, a major disadvantage of Gd-based contrast agents is low sensitivity, which limits applications to local administrations of relatively high cell quantities. This limitation is currently being approached by the development of novel T_1-contrast agents with substantially increased T_1-relaxivities (MR signal effects on T_1-weighted MR images).

Systemic injection of a contrast agent with subsequent concentration in a specific cell population would be advantageous, allowing for evaluations of stem cell transplants over a larger time window and similar workflows compared to other clinical imaging tests. MR imaging approaches are limited in this context because of the relative nonspecific in vivo distribution of clinically applicable Gd-chelates or SPIO. Targeted contrast agents or tracers that specifically accumulate in stem cell transplants after systemic administration are currently under development. For example, stem cell transplants in the spinal cord of rabbits were successfully visualized using ^{131}I-labeled transferrin injected into cerebrospinal fluid. The investigated stem cells expressed a higher level of transferrin receptors than surrounding cells and as a result concentrated radiolabeled transferrin, which allowed for the detection of the ^{131}I-enriched cells with scintigraphy.

A novel PET-based approach for imaging stem cells utilizes the FDA-approved molecular imaging probe [^{18}F]FHBG (9-[4-[^{18}F]fluoro-3-(hydroxymethyl)butyl]guanine). The PRG Herpes Simplex Virus 1 thymidine kinase (HSV1-tk) or its mutants (e.g. HSV1-sr39tk) can be delivered into stem cells by viral transduction, plasmid transfection, or electroporation/nucleofection. HSV1-sr39tk encodes the HSV1-sr39TK enzyme that catalyzes phosphorylation of [^{18}F]FHBG. The transfected stem cells can be implanted into the target tissue and/or systemically administered. At any time after implantation, the transplanted stem cells can be visualized by injecting [^{18}F]FHBG which is trapped in transplanted

stem cells, allowing for sensitive stem cell detection and quantification with PET imaging (Figure 14.2). HSV1-tk or HSV1-sr39tk can also serve as therapeutic transgenes (suicide gene) or safety genes, because cells expressing them can be killed when exposed to a pharmacological dose of antiviral drugs, ganciclovir and penciclovir.

14.2 Methods to Visualize Stem Cell Differentiation In Vivo

Although it is important to understand where stem cells migrate inside the body, of even greater interest are questions regarding the differentiation of the transplanted cells into functional target tissue. If neuronal stem cells are transplanted into the brain following an ischemic insult, what kind of cells arise? Neurons? Glial cells? Hepatocytes? To answer this question, specific characteristics of differentiated cells need to be visualized. One approach is to look for tissue-specific morphology of differentiated cells or tissue. For example, one can look for specific morphologic features of hyaline cartilage as a desired outcome of stem cell transplants into cartilage defects. However, this approach would detect complications of the engraftment process late, months or years after stem cell transplantation. In animal models, it is also possible to look for morphologic features of stem cells and their differentiated progenies. For example, neurons possess a distinct histological appearance consisting of dendrites, perikaryon, and axons, which can be recognized under a microscope, if the cells are labeled. Fluorescent microscopy observations of transplants of GFP (green fluorescent protein)-labeled neuroepithelial stem cells allowed detection of stem cell differentiation into neurons in rat brains. Unfortunately, in vivo imaging of cell histology is not clinically applicable at this time. In addition, histologic cell morphology has limited specificity, for example there is little visible difference between an embryonic stem cell and a neural stem cell.

A better way to characterize specific cell types is to take into account a cell's pattern of gene expression. Stem cells possess a different composition of expressed genes when compared to a differentiated cell. Proteins that are characteristically expressed by a specific cell population are called marker proteins. These marker proteins are fairly well characterized and can be detected with specific imaging approaches. In isolated cases, the protein that is to be imaged displays

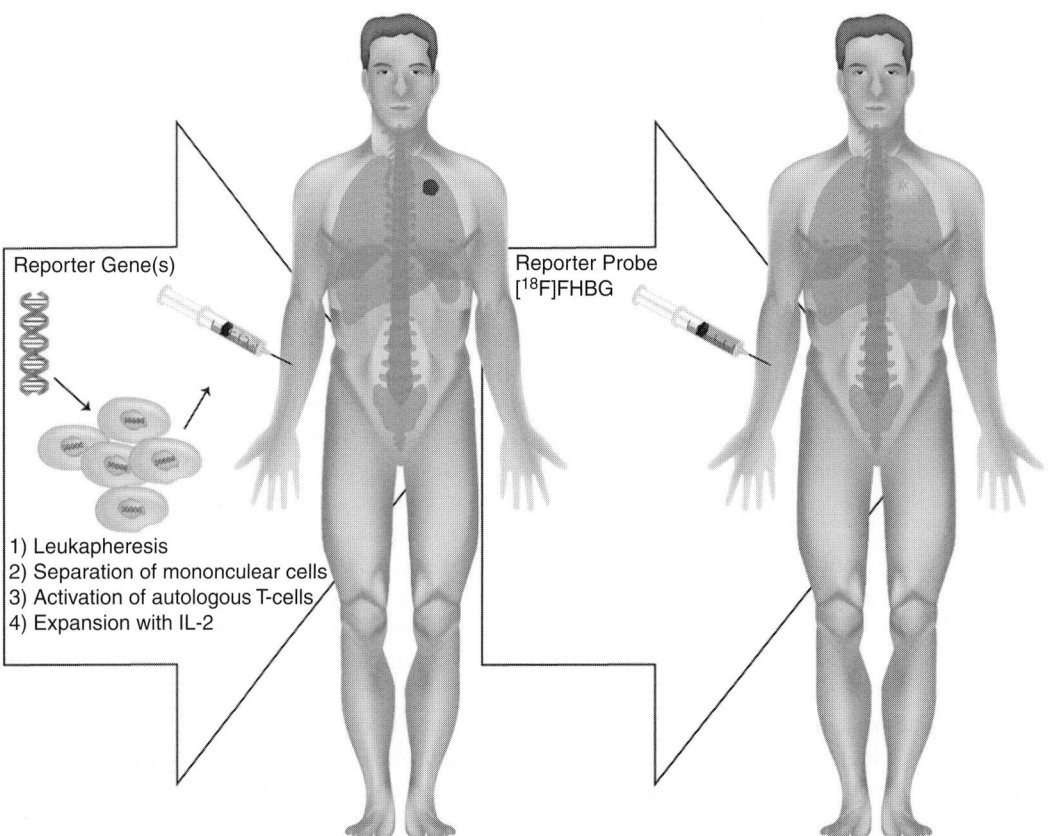

Figure 14.2 Principle of reporter gene imaging of stem cells with [^{18}F]FHBG. HSV1-sr39tk can be delivered into therapeutic stem cells by viral transduction. HSV1-sr39tk encodes the HSV1-sr39TK enzyme that can catalyze phosphorylation of [^{18}F]FHBG (9-[4-[^{18}F]fluoro-3-(hydroxymethyl) butyl]guanine). The genetically engineered therapeutic stem cells can be administered locally or intravenously (repetitively if needed). PET imaging after injection of [^{18}F]FHBG is performed before stem cell administration and at the time of desired localization of the transplanted stem cells. An increase in [^{18}F]FHBG activity at specific target sites is indicative of stem cells at that site.

inherent properties that allows it to be visualized directly. For MR imaging, this is the case with proteins related to iron metabolism, specifically ferritin and transferrin synthesis. For example, tumor cells that were genetically modified to express increased levels of transferrin caused a hypointense signal, which could be detected on T_2-weighted MR images. Most of the time, unfortunately, markers do not have these intrinsic imaging properties and molecular biology approaches are needed to visualize gene expression, for example via specific antibody-antigen interactions that can be detected with imaging techniques. Ex vivo, antibodies bound with a fluorescent dye are commonplace in histological diagnosis. In vivo, contrast agents can be bound to antibodies to visualize specific proteins. Quantum dots are novel fluorescent probes used in optical imaging. For example, quantom dots have been bound to antibodies to demonstrate detection

of Her-2, and prostate specific membrane antigen. In MR imaging, monoclonal antibodies against Her-2/neu linked to a Gd chelate successfully imaged that protein expressed on the cell membrane.

Another approach is to use the promoter of a marker and link it to a reporter gene. For example, the marker protein doublecortin could be used to visualize an an embryonic stem cell becoming a neuronal stem cell. Since doublecortin is expressed in a neuronal stem cell but not in an embryonic stem cell, the transcriptional factors that facilitate doublecortin expression must be active in a neuronal stem cell and inactive in an embryonic stem cell. If a reporter gene is placed under the promoter for doublecortin, it will only be transcribed when doublecortin is transcribed, and can be imaged with specific optical-, radiotracer-, or MR imaging approaches. While much work has been done on direct labeling and tracking of stem cells, studies for in vivo imaging of stem cell differentiation are still in a nascent stage.

14.3 Methods to Visualize Immune Responses to Stem Cell Transplants

The immune system, both innate and adaptive responses, can prevent integration of transplanted allogeneic stem cells unless the host immune system is suppressed. Similar to immune responses to solid organ transplants, transplant rejection occurs due to allelic differences in the surface antigens expressed by donor and recipient. This graft rejection must be differentiated from the nonimmune-mediated graft failure associated with inadequate stem cell numbers or stem cell apoptosis. Complex crosstalk between transplanted stem cells and host immune cells can either support tissue regeneration, for example via release of supporting cytokines, or foster an immune rejection. Like many immune responses, it is likely an acceleration of specific types of events that ultimately result in rejection. Translational approaches for noninvasive imaging of immune responses to stem cell transplants are anticipated to significantly improveour understanding of host-transplant interactions and to provide an early detection of rejection processes. This would allow earlier interventions and ultimately improve engraftment outcomes. Current clinically applicable imaging approaches allow for in vivo tracking of T-cells, dendritic cells, and macrophages.

The PET tracer fluorine-18 radiolabeled 9-b-D-arabinofuranosylguanine ($[^{18}F]$-F-AraG) is an example for imaging activated T cells and has a number of desirable characteristics. Nelarabine, a pro-drug of AraG, is approved both in the United States and Europe for treating T cell acute lymphoblastic leukemia and T cell lymphoblastic lymphoma. Inside cells, nelarabine is demethoxylated by the enzyme adenosine deaminase to AraG, which after phosphorylation by salvage pathway kinases leads to the inhibition of DNA synthesis and hence cellular cytotoxicity. AraG is processed by both mitochondrial deoxyguanosine kinase (dGK) and cytosolic deoxycytidine kinase (dCK), and both of these enzymes are highly expressed in lymphoid cells. Furthermore, AraG cytotoxicity has been shown to bc specific to T-lymphoblasts. For PET imaging, $[^{18}F]$F-AraG is administered in tracer doses several thousandfold less than pharmacological doses and should not be cytotoxic to any cell. Most importantly, in preliminary cell culture studies, a significant four fold higher accumulation of $[^{18}F]$F-AraG was found in activated primary mouse T cells versus naïve primary mouse T cells. T cells can be tracked in vivo with $[^{18}F]$F-AraG in order to detect acute transplant rejection.

Macrophages also play a major role in transplant rejection processes, in addition to antigen-presenting dendritic cells, activated Tcells, and a variety of other leukocyte subpopulations. Macrophages can be visualized in stem cell transplants using MR imaging and the FDA-approved iron supplement ferumoxytol (Feraheme) as a cell marker. Ferumoxytol is composed of nanoparticles with a hydrodynamic diameter of 20–30 nm, an iron oxide core, and a carboxydextran coat. Ferumoxytol can be used "off label" as an MR contrast agent; it provides strong T1- and T2-enhancement on MR images. Upon intravenous injection, ferumoxytol nanoparticles initially distribute in the blood pool, then they slowly extravasate into the interstitium of extracerebral organs, where they are phagocytosed by macrophages. Ferumoxytol can detect and quantify differential macrophage infiltrations in tumors and stem cell transplants on MR images and has been shown to be safe in in patients with renal insufficiency. Macrophage migration into stem cell transplants can be visualized by "prelabeling" macrophages in the reticuloendothelial system (RES) with intravenous ferumoxytol prior to a stem cell transplant. Once RES cells are labeled, (unlabeled) stem cells are transplanted. A migration of the labeled macrophages into stem cell transplants can then be visualized with MR imaging (Figure 14.3).

Immune cell tracking techniques may enable us to overcome the bottleneck of diagnosing stem cell transplant rejection early after transplantation, avoiding long-term and invasive follow-up studies of lost transplants, and help in assigning patients with transplant rejection to early interventions or alternative treatment options. Potential further applications include comparative in vivo investigations of the host immune response to different stem cell types (hESC, hMSC, hiPS); comparisons of autologous and allogeneic transplants; investigations of genetically engineered stem cells; comparisons of different scaffolds and growth factors; and assessments of demographic effects on stem cell engraftment outcomes. Significant improvement and acceleration of the development of successful therapies for tissue regeneration in patients could be achieved by exploiting novel, immediately

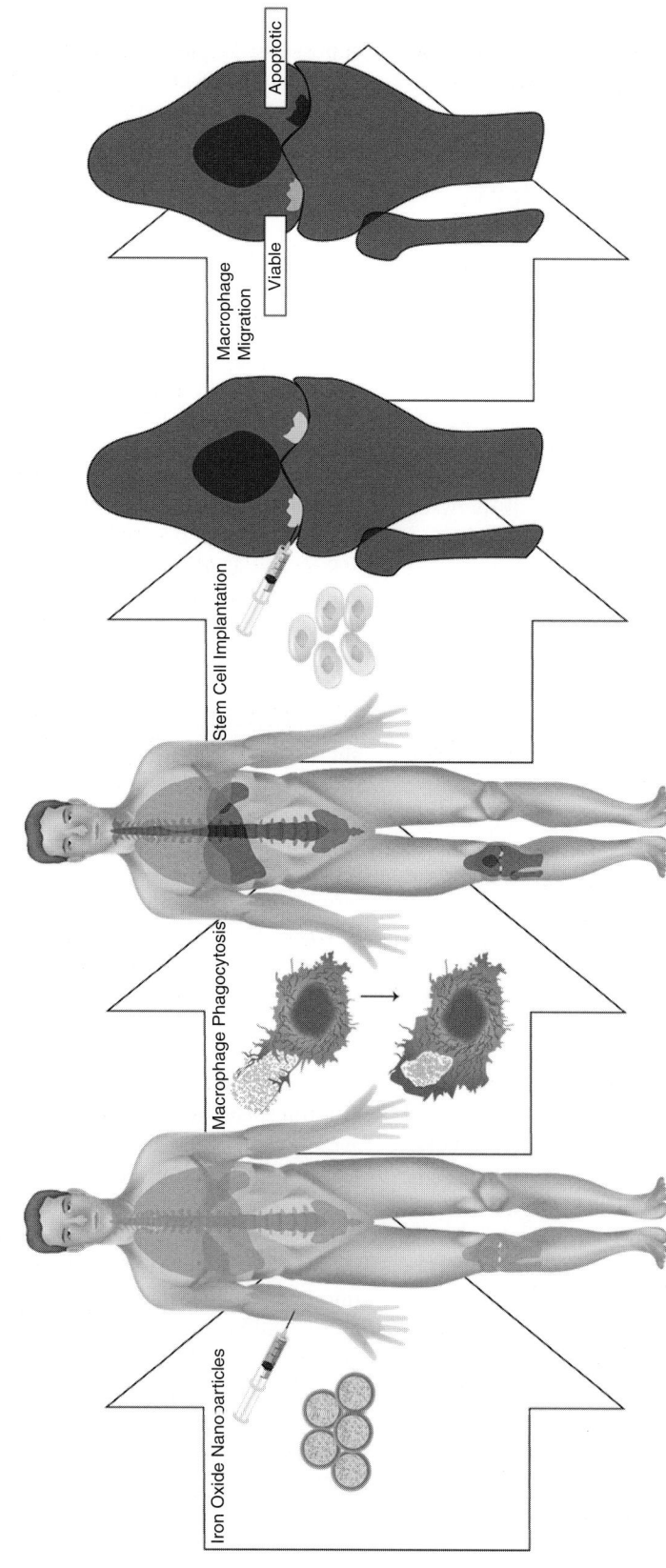

Figure 14.3 Principle of pre-labeling macrophages in the reticuloethothelial system with intravenously injected iron oxide nanoparticles, followed by stem cell transplants into osteochondral defects of a knee joint. A migration of iron oxide labeled macrophages into the stem cell transplant can be diagnosed by negative (dark) signal effects on T2-weighted MR images, indicating transplant rejection or failure.

clinically applicable imaging techniques as a new, critical non-invasive tool to monitor stem cell engraftment outcomes.

Further Reading

1. Bursac, N. Stem cell therapies for heart disease: why do we need bioengineers? *IEEE Eng Med Biol Mag* 26, 76–79 (2007).

2. Christoforou, N. & Gearhart, J.D. Stem cells and their potential in cell-based cardiac therapies. *Prog Cardiovasc Dis* 49, 396–413 (2007).

3. Mimeault, M., Hauke, R. & Batra, S.K. Stem cells: a revolution in therapeutics-recent advances in stem cell biology and their therapeutic applications in regenerative medicine and cancer therapies. *Clin Pharmacol Ther* 82, 252–264 (2007).

4. Vawda, R., Woodbury, J., Covey, M., Levison, S.W. & Mehmet, H. Stem cell therapies for perinatal brain injuries. *Semin Fetal Neonatal Med* 12, 259–272 (2007).

5. Adler, R. Curing blindness with stem cells: hope, reality, and challenges. *Adv Exp Med Biol* 613, 3–20 (2008).

6. Madan, B. & Schey, S.A. Reversible cortical blindness and convulsions with cyclosporin A toxicity in a patient undergoing allogeneic peripheral stem cell transplantation. *Bone Marrow Transplant* 20, 793–795 (1997).

7. Mays, R.W., van't Hof, W., Ting, A.E., Perry, R. & Deans, R. Development of adult pluripotent stem cell therapies for ischemic injury and disease. *Expert Opin Biol Ther* 7, 173–184 (2007).

8. Cizkova, D. Kakinohana, O., Kurcharova, K., Marsala, S., Johe, K., Hazel, T., Functional recovery in rats with ischemic paraplegia after spinal grafting of human spinal stem cells. *Neuroscience* 147, 546–560 (2007).

9. Mummery, C.L. & van Laake, L.W. Progress and clashes in stem cell therapy research. *Ned Tijdschr Geneeskd* 150, 943–947 (2006).

10. Mabed, M. & Shahin, M. Mesenchymal stem cell-based therapy for the treatment of type 1 diabetes mellitus. *Curr Stem Cell Res Ther* 7, 179–190 (2012).

11. Dupont, K.M., Sharma, K., Stevens, H.Y., Boerckel, J.D., García, A.J., Guldberg, R.E., et al. Human stem cell delivery for treatment of large segmental bone defects. *Proc Natl Acad Sci U S A* 107, 3305–3310 (2010).

12. Qi, Y., Feng, G. & Yan, W. Mesenchymal stem cell-based treatment for cartilage defects in osteoarthritis. *Mol Biol Rep* 39, 5683–5689 (2012).

13. Sutton, E.J., Henning, T.D., Pichler, B.J., Bremer, C. & Daldrup-Link, H.E. Cell tracking with optical imaging. *Eur Radiol* 18, 2021–2032 (2008).

14. Galle, J., Bader, A., Hepp, P., Grill, W., Fuchs, B., et al. Mesenchymal stem cells in cartilage repair: state of the art and methods to monitor cell growth, differentiation and cartilage regeneration. *Curr Med Chem* 17, 2274–2291 (2010).

15. Omlor, G.W., Bertram, H., Kleinschmidt, K., Fischer, J., Brohm, K., Guehring, T., et al. Methods to monitor distribution and metabolic activity of mesenchymal stem cells following in vivo injection into nucleotomized porcine intervertebral discs. *Eur Spine J* 19, 601–612 (2010).

16. Jing, M., Liu, X.Q., Liang, P., Li, C.Y., Zhang, X.T., Wang, D., et al. Labeling neural stem cells with superparamagnetic iron oxide in vitro and tracking after implantation with MRI in vivo. *Zhonghua Yi Xue Za Zhi* 84, 1386–1389 (2004).

17. Narayanan, R., Tare, N.S., Benjamin, W.R. & Gubler, U. A sensitive technique to monitor gene transfer and expression in bone marrow stem cells. *Exp Hematol* 17, 832–835 (1989).

18. Togel, F., Yang, Y., Zhang, P., Hu, Z. & Westenfelder, C. Bioluminescence imaging to monitor the in vivo distribution of administered mesenchymal stem cells in acute kidney injury. *Am J Physiol Renal Physiol* 295, F315–321 (2008).

19. Kouris, K. & Jackson, D.F. Effects of radioactive decay and their implications on in vivo metabolic imaging. *Am J Physiol Imaging* 2, 44–47 (1987).

20. Su, J.L., Wang, B., Wilson, K.E., Bayer, C.L., Chen, Y.S., Kim, S., et al. Advances in Clinical and Biomedical Applications of Photoacoustic Imaging. *Expert Opin Med Diagn* 4, 497–510 (2010).

21. Kitai, T., Torii, M., Sugie, T., Kanao, S., Mikami, Y., Shiina, T., et al. Photoacoustic mammography: initial clinical results. *Breast Cancer* 21, 146–153 (2012).

22. Su, J., Karpiouk, A., Wang, B. & Emelianov, S. Photoacoustic imaging of clinical metal needles in tissue. *J Biomed Opt* 15, 021309 (2010).

23. Jokerst, J.V., Thangaraj, M., Kempen, P.J., Sinclair, R. & Gambhir, S.S. Photoacoustic imaging of mesenchymal stem cells in living mice via silica-coated gold Nanorods. *ACS Nano* 6, 5920–5930 (2012).

24. Wang, C., Cheng, L., Xu, H. & Liu, Z. Towards whole-body imaging at the single cell level using ultra-sensitive stem cell labeling with oligo-arginine modified upconversion nanoparticles. *Biomaterials* 33, 4872–4881 (2012).

25. Lee, J.H., Jung, M.J., Hwang, Y.H., Lee, Y.J., Lee, S., et al. Heparin-coated superparamagnetic iron oxide for

in vivo MR imaging of human MSCs. *Biomaterials* 33, 4861–4871 (2012).

26. Sykova, E., Jendelova, P. & Herynek, V. Magnetic resonance imaging of stem cell migration. *Methods Mol Biol* 750, 79–90 (2011).

27. Henning, T.D., Saborowski, O., Golovko, D., Boddington, S., Bauer, J.S., Gu, Y., et al. Cell labeling with the positive MR contrast agent Gadofluorine M. *Eur Radiol* 17, 1226–1234 (2007).

28. Nejadnik H.T., Do, T., Sutton, E.J., Baehner, F., Horvai, A., Sennino, B., et al. MR imaging features of gadofluorine labeled matrix associated stem cell implants in cartilage defects. *PLoS One* 7, e49971 (2012).

29. Daldrup-Link, H.E., Rudelius, M., Pointek, G., Metz, S., Brauer, R., et al. Migration of iron oxide-labeled human hematopoietic progenitor cells in a mouse model: in vivo monitoring with 1.5-T MR imaging equipment. *Radiology* 234, 197–205 (2005).

30. Henning T.D., Boddington, S., Taubert, S., Jha, P., Tavri, S., Golovko, D., Ackermann, L. & Daldrup-Link, H.E. Somatic differentiation and MR imaging of magnetically labeled human embryonic stem cells. *Cell Transplantation* (2012).

31. Henning, T.D., Gawande, R., Khurana, A., Tavri, S., Mandrussow, L., Golovko, D., et al. Magnetic resonance imaging of ferumoxide-labeled mesenchymal stem cells in cartilage defects: in vitro and in vivo investigations. *Mol Imaging* 11, 197–209 (2012).

32. Chung, J. & Yang, P.C. Molecular Imaging of Stem Cell Transplantation in Myocardial Disease. *Curr Cardiovasc Imaging Rep* 3, 106–112 (2010).

33. Khurana, N.H., Gawande, R., Lin, G., Lee, S., Messing, S., Castaneda, R., Derugin, N., Pisani, L., Lue, T.F., & Daldrup-Link, H.E. Intravenous ferumoxytol allows non-invasive MR imaging monitoring of macrophage migration into stem cell transplants. *Radiology* (2012).

34. Rinck, P.A. *Magnetic Resonance in Medicine: The Basic Textbook of the European Magnetic Resonance Forum* (Blackwell Scientific Publications: Oxford; Boston, 1993).

35. Castaneda, R.T., Khurana, A., Khan, R. & Daldrup-Link, H.E. Labeling stem cells with ferumoxytol, an FDA-approved iron oxide nanoparticle. *J Vis Exp*, e3482 (2011).

36. Castaneda, R.T., Boddington, S., Henning, T.D., Wendland, M., Mandrussow, Liu, S., et al. Labeling human embryonic stem-cell-derived cardiomyocytes for tracking with MR imaging. *Pediatr Radiol* 41, 1384–1392 (2011).

37. van Buul, G.M., Kotek, G., Wielopolski, P.A., Farrell, E., Bos, P.K., Weinans, H., et al. Clinically translatable cell tracking and quantification by MRI in cartilage repair using superparamagnetic iron oxides. *PLoS One* 6, e17001 (2011).

38. Sykova, E. & Jendelova, P. In vivo tracking of stem cells in brain and spinal cord injury. *Prog Brain Res* 161, 367–383 (2007).

39. Bernsen, M.R., Moelker, A.D., Wielopolski, P.A., van Tiel, S.T. & Krestin, G.P. Labelling of mammalian cells for visualisation by MRI. *Eur Radiol* 20, 255–274 (2010).

40. Tseng, C.L., Shih, I.L., Stobinski, L. & Lin, F.H. Gadolinium hexanedione nanoparticles for stem cell labeling and tracking via magnetic resonance imaging. *Biomaterials* 31, 5427–5435 (2010).

41. Hsiao, J.K., Tsai, C.P., Chung, T.H., Hung, Y., Yao, M., Liu, H.M., et al. Mesoporous silica nanoparticles as a delivery system of gadolinium for effective human stem cell tracking. *Small* 4, 1445–1452 (2008).

42. Vuu, K., Xie, J., McDonald, M.A., Bernardo, M., Hunter, F., Zhang, Y., et al. Gadolinium-rhodamine nanoparticles for cell labeling and tracking via magnetic resonance and optical imaging. *Bioconjug Chem* 16, 995–999 (2005).

43. Schroder, U., Segrern, S., Gemmefors, C., Hedlund, G., Jansson, B., Sjögren, H.O., et al. Magnetic carbohydrate nanoparticles for affinity cell separation. *J Immunol Methods* 93, 45–53 (1986).

44. Kircher, M.F., Gambhir, S.S. & Grimm, J. Noninvasive cell-tracking methods. *Nat Rev Clin Oncol* 8, 677–688 (2011).

45. Guenoun, J., Koning, G.A., Doeswijk, G., Bosman, L., Wieloposki, P.A., Krestin, G.P., et al. Cationic Gd-DTPA liposomes for highly efficient labeling of mesenchymal stem cells and cell tracking with MRI. *Cell Transplant* 21, 191–205 (2012).

46. Shen, J., Duan, X.H., Cheng, L.N., Zhong, X.M., Guo, R.M., Zhang, F., et al. In vivo MR imaging tracking of transplanted mesenchymal stem cells in a rabbit model of acute peripheral nerve traction injury. *J Magn Reson Imaging* 32, 1076–1085 (2010).

47. Anderson, S.A., Lee, K.K. & Frank, J.A. Gadolinium-fullerenol as a paramagnetic contrast agent for cellular imaging. *Invest Radiol* 41, 332–338 (2006).

48. Caravan, P. Strategies for increasing the sensitivity of gadolinium based MRI contrast agents. *Chem Soc Rev* 35, 512–523 (2006).

49. Uysal, E., Erturk, S.M., Yildirim, H., Seleker, F. & Basak, M. Sensitivity of immediate and delayed gadolinium-enhanced MRI after injection of 0.5 M and 1.0 M gadolinium chelates for detecting multiple sclerosis lesions. *AJR Am J Roentgenol* 188, 697–702 (2007).

50. Raymond, K.N. & Pierre, V.C. Next generation, high relaxivity gadolinium MRI agents. *Bioconjug Chem* 16, 3–8 (2005).

51. Haar, P.J., Broaddus, W.C., Chen, Z.J., Fatouros, P.P., Gillies, G.T., Corwin, F.D., et al. Gd-DTPA T1 relaxivity in brain tissue obtained by convection-enhanced delivery, magnetic resonance imaging and emission spectroscopy. *Phys Med Biol* 55, 3451–3465 (2010).

52. Goswami, L.N., White, W.H. 3rd, Spemyak, J.A., Ethirajan, M., Chen, Y., Missert, J.R., et al. Synthesis of Tumor-avid Photosensitizer-Gd(III)DTPA conjugates: impact of the number of gadolinium units in T1/T2 relaxivity, intracellular localization, and photosensitizing efficacy. *Bioconjug Chem* 21, 816–827 (2010).

53. Park, J.Y., Baek, M.J., Choi, E.S., Woo, S., Kim, J.H., Kim, T.J., et al. Paramagnetic ultrasmall gadolinium oxide nanoparticles as advanced T1 MRI contrast agent: account for large longitudinal relaxivity, optimal particle diameter, and in vivo T1 MR images. *ACS Nano* 3, 3663–3669 (2009).

54. Caravan, P., Farrar, C.T., Frullano, L. & Uppal, R. Influence of molecular parameters and increasing magnetic field strength on relaxivity of gadolinium- and manganese-based T1 contrast agents. *Contrast Media Mol Imaging* 4, 89–100 (2009).

55. Ding, W.M., Tian, J.H., Bai, J.Z. & Shen, L. Transferrin receptor imaging for tracing mesenchymal stem cells implanted in the spinal cord. *Nan Fang Yi Ke Da Xue Xue Bao* 27, 1318–1322 (2007).

56. Bai, J.Z., Ding, W.M., Liu, Z.J., Yu, M.J., Tian, J.H., Wang, F., et al. Transferrin receptor expression of human mesenchymal stem cells and in vitro tracking by autoradiography after transplantation in spinal cord. *Beijing Da Xue Xue Bao* 36, 276–280 (2004).

57. Bai, J., Ding, W., Yu, M., Du, J., Liu, Z., Jia, B., et al. Radionuclide imaging of mesenchymal stem cells transplanted into spinal cord. *Neuroreport* 15, 1117–1120 (2004).

58. Ding, W., Bai, J., Zhang, J., Chen, Y., Cao, L., He, Y., et al. In vivo tracking of implanted stem cells using radio-labeled transferrin scintigraphy. *Nucl Med Biol* 31, 719–725 (2004).

59. Johnson, M., Karanikolas, B.D., Priceman, S.J., Powell, R., Black, M.E., Wu, H.M., et al. Titration of variant HSV1-tk gene expression to determine the sensitivity of 18F-FHBG PET imaging in a prostate tumor. *J Nucl Med* 50, 757–764 (2009).

60. Najjar, A.M., Nishii, R., Maxwell, D.S., Volgin, A., Mukhopadhyay, U., Bommann, W.G., et al. Molecular-genetic PET imaging using an HSV1-tk mutant reporter gene with enhanced specificity to acycloguanosine nucleoside analogs. *J Nucl Med* 50, 409–416 (2009).

61. Roelants, V., Labar, D., de Meester, C., Havaux, X., Tabilio, A., Gambhir, S.S., et al. Comparison between adenoviral and retroviral vectors for the transduction of the thymidine kinase PET reporter gene in rat mesenchymal stem cells. *J Nucl Med* 49, 1836–1844 (2008).

62. Chang, G.Y., Cao, F., Krishnan, M., Huang, M., Li, Z., Xie, X., et al. Positron emission tomography imaging of conditional gene activation in the heart. *J Mol Cell Cardiol* 43, 18–26 (2007).

63. Yaghoubi, S.S. & Gambhir, S.S. PET imaging of herpes simplex virus type 1 thymidine kinase (HSV1-tk) or mutant HSV1-sr39tk reporter gene expression in mice and humans using [18F]FHBG. *Nat Protoc* 1, 3069–3075 (2006).

64. Yaghoubi, S.S., Couto, M.A., Chen, C.C., Polavaram, L., Cui, G., Sen, L., et al. Preclinical safety evaluation of 18F-FHBG: a PET reporter probe for imaging herpes simplex virus type 1 thymidine kinase (HSV1-tk) or mutant HSV1-sr39tk's expression. *J Nucl Med* 47, 706–715 (2006).

65. Yaghoubi, S.S., Barrio, J.R., Namavari, M., Satyamurthy, N., Phelps, M.E., Herschman, H.R., et al. Imaging progress of herpes simplex virus type 1 thymidine kinase suicide gene therapy in living subjects with positron emission tomography. *Cancer Gene Ther* 12, 329–339 (2005).

66. 9-(4-[18F]Fluoro-3-hydroxymethylbutyl)guanine. in *Molecular Imaging and Contrast Agent Database (MICAD)* (Bethesda (MD), 2004).

67. 2′-Deoxy-2′-[18F]fluoro-5-fluoro-1-beta-D-arabinofuranosyluracil. in *Molecular Imaging and Contrast Agent Database (MICAD)* (Bethesda (MD), 2004).

68. 2′-Fluoro-2′-deoxy-5′-[124I]iodo-1beta-d-arabinofuranosyluracil. in *Molecular Imaging and Contrast Agent Database (MICAD)* (Bethesda (MD), 2004).

69. Tang, G., Tang, X., Li, H., Wang, M., Li, B., Liang, M., et al. A simplified one-pot automated synthesis of [18F]FHBG for imaging reporter gene expression. *Nucl Med Commun* 31, 211–216 (2010).

70. Green, L.A., Nguyen, K., Berenji, B., Iyer, M., Bauer, E., Barrio, J.R., et al. A tracer kinetic model for 18F-FHBG for quantitating herpes simplex virus type 1 thymidine kinase reporter gene expression in living animals using PET. *J Nucl Med* 45, 1560–1570 (2004).

71. Uchida, K., Momiyama, T., Okano, H., Yuzaki, M., Koizumi, A., Mine, Y., et al. Potential functional neural repair with grafted neural stem cells of early embryonic neuroepithelial origin. *Neurosci Res* 52, 276–286 (2005).

72. Rudelius, M., Daldrup-Link, H.E., Heinzmann, U., Piontek, G., Settles, M., Link, T.M., et al. Highly efficient paramagnetic labelling of embryonic and neuronal stem cells. *Eur J Nucl Med Mol Imaging* 30, 1038–1044 (2003).

73. Weissleder, R., Moore, A., Mahmood, U., Bhorade, R., Benveniste, H., Chiocca, E.A., et al. In vivo magnetic resonance imaging of transgene expression. *Nat Med* 6, 351–355 (2000).

74. Jiang, W., Papa, E., Fischer, H., Mardyani, S. & Chan, W.C. Semiconductor quantum dots as contrast agents for whole animal imaging. *Trends Biotechnol* 22, 607–609 (2004).

75. Wu, X., Liu, H., Liu, J., Haley, K.N., Treasway, J.A., Larson, J.P., et al. Immunofluorescent labeling of cancer marker Her2 and other cellular targets with semiconductor quantum dots. *Nat Biotechnol* 21, 41–46 (2003).

76. Gao, Y., Stanford, W.L. & Chan, W.C. Quantum-dot-encoded microbeads for multiplexed genetic detection of non-amplified DNA samples. *Small* 7, 137–146 (2011).

77. Artemov, D. Molecular magnetic resonance imaging with targeted contrast agents. *J Cell Biochem* 90, 518–524 (2003).

78. Couillard-Despres, S., Quehl, E., Altendorfer, K., Karl, C., Ploetz, S., Bogdahn, U., et al. Human in vitro reporter model of neuronal development and early differentiation processes. *BMC Neurosci* 9, 31 (2008).

79. Karl, C., Couillard-Despres, S., Prang, P., Munding, M., Kilb, W., Brigadski, T., et al. Neuronal precursor-specific activity of a human doublecortin regulatory sequence. *J Neurochem* 92, 264–282 (2005).

80. Heng, B.C., Liu, H. & Cao, T. Transplanted human embryonic stem cells as biological 'catalysts' for tissue repair and regeneration. *Med Hypotheses* 64, 1085–1088 (2005).

81. Wang, Z., Yang, Z., He, X. & Tu, J. Aggrecanases gene inhibition in chondrocytes: a new possible strategy to relieve immune rejection of transplants. *Med Hypotheses* 72, 196–198 (2009).

82. Bazyar, N., Azarpira, N., Khatami, S.R., Galehdari, H. & Salahi, H. Complement C3 gene polymorphism in renal transplantation (an Iranian experience). *Gene* 498, 254–258 (2012).

83. Cao, T.M., Lo, B., Ranheim, E.A., Grumet, F.C. & Shizuru, J.A. Variable hematopoietic graft rejection and graft-versus-host disease in MHC-matched strains of mice. *Proc Natl Acad Sci U S A* 100, 11571–11576 (2003).

84. Daldrup-Link, H.E., Rudelius, M., Oostendorp, R.A., Jacobs, V.R., Simon, G.H., Gooding, C., et al. Comparison of iron oxide labeling properties of hematopoietic progenitor cells from umbilical cord blood and from peripheral blood for subsequent in vivo tracking in a xenotransplant mouse model XXX. *Acad Radiol* 12, 502–510 (2005).

85. Yaghoubi, S.S., Jensen, M.C., Satyamurthy, N., Budhiraja, S., Paik, D., Czernin, J., et al. Noninvasive detection of therapeutic cytolytic T cells with 18F-FHBG PET in a patient with glioma. *Nat Clin Pract Oncol* 6, 53–58 (2009).

86. Kutschka, I., Chen, I.Y., Kofidis, T., von Dedenfeld, G., Sheikh, A.Y., Hendry, S.L., et al. In vivo optical bioluminescence imaging of collagen-supported cardiac cell grafts. *J Heart Lung Transplant* 26, 273–280 (2007).

87. Lee, S.W., Padmanabhan, P., Ray, P., Gambhir, S.S., Doyle, T., Contag, C., et al. Stem cell-mediated accelerated bone healing observed with in vivo molecular and small animal imaging technologies in a model of skeletal injury. *J Orthop Res* 27, 295–302 (2009).

88. Tavare, R., Sagoo, P., Varama, G., Tanriver, Y., Warely, A., Diebold, S.S., et al. Monitoring of in vivo function of superparamagnetic iron oxide labelled murine dendritic cells during anti-tumour vaccination. *PLoS One* 6, e19662 (2011).

89. Namavari, M., Chag, Y.F., Kusler, B., Yaghoubi, S., Mitchell, B.S., Gambhir, S.S., et al. Synthesis of 2'-deoxy-2'-[18F]fluoro-9-beta-D-arabinofuranosylguanine: a novel agent for imaging T-cell activation with PET. *Mol Imaging Biol* 13, 812–818 (2011).

90. Curbo, S. & Karlsson, A. Nelarabine: a new purine analog in the treatment of hematologic malignancies. *Rev Recent Clin Trials* 1, 185–192 (2006).

91. Leanza, L., Miazzi, C., Ferraro, P., Reichard, P. & Bianchi, V. Activation of guanine-beta-D-arabinofuranoside and deoxyguanosine to triphosphates by a common pathway blocks T lymphoblasts at different checkpoints. *Exp Cell Res* 316, 3443–3453 (2010).

92. Spasokoukotskaja, T., Amer, E.S., Brosjo, O., Gunven, P., Juliusson, G., Liliemark, J., et al. Expression of deoxycytidine kinase and phosphorylation of 2-chlorodeoxyadenosine in human normal and tumour cells and tissues. *Eur J Cancer* 31A, 202–208 (1995).

93. Zhu, C., Johansson, M. & Karlsson, A. Differential incorporation of 1-beta-D-arabinofuranosylcytosine and 9-beta-D-arabinofuranosylguanine into nuclear and mitochondrial DNA. *FEBS Lett* 474, 129–132 (2000).

94. Zhu, C., Johansson, M. & Karlsson, A. Incorporation of nucleoside analogs into nuclear or mitochondrial DNA is determined by the intracellular phosphorylation site. *J Biol Chem* 275, 26727–26731 (2000).

95. Hamilton, B.E., Nesbit, G.M., Dosa, E., Gahramanov, S., Rooney, B., Nesbit, E.G., et al. Comparative analysis of ferumoxytol and gadoteridol enhancement using T1- and T2-weighted MRI in neuroimaging. *AJR Am J Roentgenol* 197, 981–988 (2011).

96. Thu, M.S., Bryant, L.H., Coppola, T., Jordan, E.K., Budde, M.D., Lewis, B.K., et al. Self-assembling nanocomplexes by combining ferumoxytol, heparin and protamine for cell tracking by magnetic resonance imaging. *Nat Med* 18, 463–467 (2012).

97. Daldrup-Link, H.E., Golovko, D., Ruffell, B., Denardo, D.G., Castaneda, R., Ansari, C., et al. MRI of tumor-associated macrophages with clinically applicable iron oxide nanoparticles. *Clin Cancer Res* 17, 5695–5704 (2011).

98. Lu, M., Cohen, M.H., Rieves, D. & Pazdur, R. FDA report: Ferumoxytol for intravenous iron therapy in adult patients with chronic kidney disease. *Am J Hematol* 85, 315–319 (2010).

Amyloid Imaging

Heather Jacene

15.1 Introduction

Amyloid is protein composed of linear nonbranching fibrils arranged in sheets. Amyloidosis is a disease characterized by misfolding proteins, aggregation, and extracellular depositions of amyloid in tissue and organs. There are at least 20 described types of amyloid protein in humans which vary by precursor protein and resultant organs of deposition. Amyloid deposition may be localized (e.g. brain in Alzheimer's disease (AD)) or systemic (e.g. primary light chain amyloidosis), and there is a wide range of clinical manifestations, from none to severe organ dysfunction.

In regard to selective imaging of amyloid protein, most work thus far has been on developing agents targeting beta (β)-amyloid (Aβ) plaques in the brain, which will be the focus of this chapter. Clinical applications for amyloid imaging of the heart and systemic amyloid deposition are also emerging.

15.2 Beta Amyloid Plaques and Pathologic Basis for Alzheimer's Disease

Aβ protein is a 36–43 amino acid peptide cleaved from the transmembrane Aβ protein precursor by β and gamma (γ) sectretase (Figure 15.1). The normal function of Aβ protein is not well understood. Some described potential roles are activation of kinase enzymes, protection against oxidative stress, regulation of cholesterol transport, and serving as a transcription factor or antimicrobial. Plaques containing Aβ protein are described as diffuse or dense, with current imaging probes having affinity for the latter.

15.3 Radiopharmaceuticals for Aβ Amyloid PET Imaging

15.3.1 Carbon-11 Pittsburgh Complex B

Carbon-11 Pittsburgh (^{11}C-PiB) was the first radiopharmaceutical developed for targeting Aβ plaques.

[11]C-PiB is derived from thioflavin T, a fluorescent dye that binds amyloid and is used to histologically identify plaques in brain tissue specimens. PET imaging is performed 40–50 minutes after tracer injection for 20–30 minutes. Normal distribution of ^{11}C-PiB is in cerebral white matter (Figure 15.2, top row). In disease states, there is usually much less dense plaque deposition in cerebellar gray matter compared to cortical gray matter, so the cerebellum is most commonly used as a reference region. Visually, uptake of ^{11}C-PiB in cortical gray matter at least equal to or greater than white matter is considered abnormal (Figure 15.2, bottom row). Standardized uptake value (SUV) ratios comparing cortical to cerebellar gray matter uptake may also be determined, with the upper limit of normal reported as 1.3–1.6. Correlations between ^{11}C-PiB uptake in cortical gray matter and postmortem assessments of Aβ plaques have been demonstrated.

15.3.2 Fluorine-18 Labeled Amyloid Imaging Agents

As with all ^{11}C labeled radiopharmaceticals, the short 20-minute half-life of ^{11}C is a major limitation for widespread use, requiring an on-site (or nearby) cyclotron. Consequently, several fluorine-18 (^{18}F)-labeled radiotracers for Aβ amyloid imaging have been developed. ^{18}F-florbetepir is the first to be approved by the Food and Drug Administration and others being evaluated in clinical trials include ^{18}F-flutemetamol, ^{18}F-florbetaben, and ^{18}F-NAV4694. ^{18}F-florbetepir uptake on PET imaging has been shown to correlate with the presence and quantity of Aβ amyloid at autopsy.

PET imaging is obtained for 15–20 minutes, approximately 50 minutes after the injection of ^{18}F-florbetepir and 80–90 minutes after the administration of ^{18}F-flutemetamol and ^{18}F-florbetaben. Normal uptake in white matter is higher for the ^{18}F-labeled

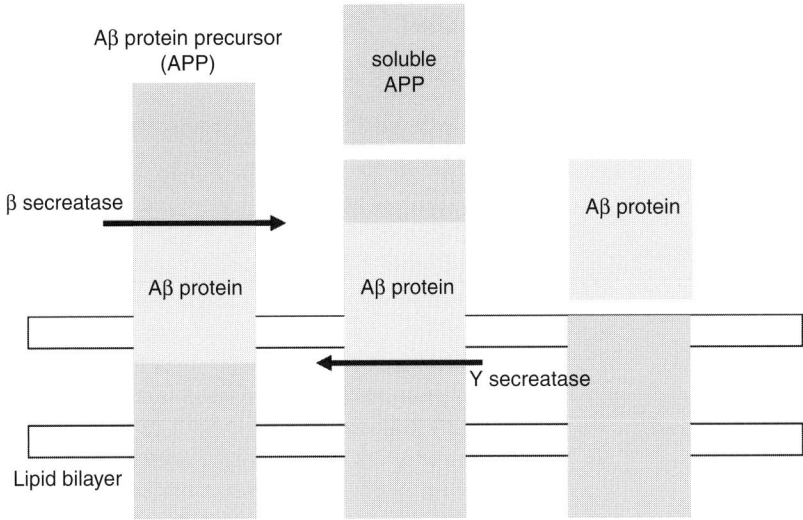

Figure 15.1 Cleavage of Aβ protein precursor to Aβ protein
Alzheimer's disease (AD) is characterized microscopically by widespread cellular degeneration and an excess of neuritic plaques (i.e. dense plaques that cause neuronal damage and inflammation) and cytoplasmic neurofibrillary tangles in the brain. Aβ protein is the most abundant component of the neuritic plaques and these dense plaques are predominantly found in the frontal cortex, cingulated gyrus, precuneus, lateral parietal, and temporal regions in AD. The excess of Aβ protein has been postulated to be due to reduced breakdown or increased production.

agents compared to ^{11}C-PiB (Figure 15.3A). Uptake of ^{18}F-labeled agents in the cortex in AD, therefore, may be equal to or less than that of white matter. On a negative scan, there is a clear distinction between gray and white matter whereas on a positive scan, there is loss of the clear gray-white distinction (Figure 15.3B).

15.3.3 Technique for Interpretation of Brain Amyloid PET Imaging

A common approach has been suggested for reading brain amyloid PET with ^{11}C-PiB and the ^{18}F-labeled agents. The general steps are: (1) set an optimal dynamic color or black and white range using cerebellar gray matter as a reference; (2) review the mid-sagittal plane for uptake in the orbitofrontal cortex, precuneous and posterior cingulated gyri; (3) review the transaxial slices for uptake in the frontal, temporal, parietal, occipital, and striatal regions. Normal and abnormal findings are described in the previous sections.

Pitfalls for interpretation include patient motion, partial volume effects from atrophy, obliquing slicing through white matter (causing a false positive) due to improper orientation for reconstruction. The CT obtained for attenuation correction is often helpful for recognizing these pitfalls.

15.4 Clinical Applications of Brain Aβ Amyloid PET Imaging

AD is the most common type of dementia and is characterized clinically by progressive memory loss and cognitive decline in one other area to the point that activities of daily life are affected. The diagnosis of AD is based on clinical presentation with findings on imaging studies and laboratory investigations providing adjunctive information. The major differential diagnoses for AD are vascular, frontotemporal, and Lewy body dementia. Mild cognitive impairment (MCI) is a milder form of cognitive decline that does not affect activities of daily life. MCI may progress to AD; however, about 30–40 percent of the time it does not progress and in 20 percent of cases it progresses to another type of dementia.

Appropriate Use Criteria for Amyloid PET imaging of the brain were published in 2013. The major indications for amyloid PET imaging are to distinguish possible AD from other types of dementia, to evaluate persistent or progressive unexplained MCI,

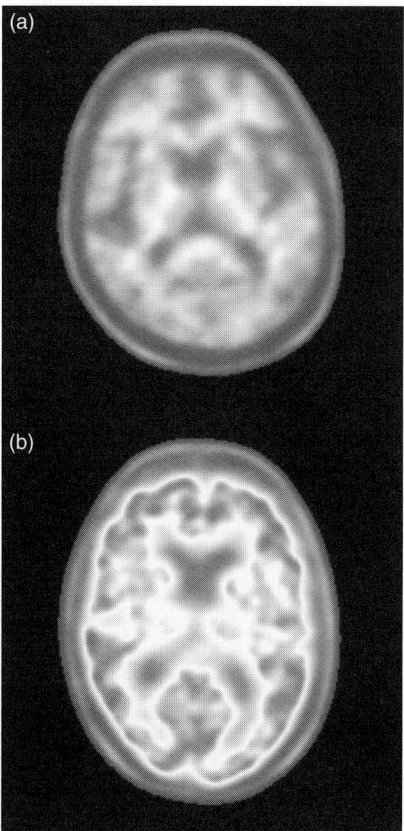

Figure 15.2 Normal ¹¹C-PiB PET Images (top row) in a healthy control (HC) show mild uptake in white matter. **Abnormal ¹¹C-PiB PET Images** (bottom row) in a patient with Alzheimer's dementia (AD) show uptake in gray matter that is greater than white matter. Reprinted with permission from Ng et al. Visual Assessment versus Quantitative Assessment of ¹¹C-PIB PET and ¹⁸F-FDG PET for Detection of Alzheimer's Disease. *J Nucl Med* 2007; 48:547–52.

and to evaluate progressive dementia of early onset (age less than 65) in patients with objective measures of cognitive decline and in whom knowledge of Aβ pathology will alter management.

Aβ plaques are not present in frontotemporal dementia (FTD), and amyloid imaging has been reported to differentiate FTD from AD with high accuracy. However, amyloid imaging cannot distinguish AD from Lewy body dementia or cerebral amyloid angiopathy. In addition, the accuracy of ¹¹C-PiB amyloid imaging decreases with age due to the increasing prevalence of Aβ plaques/AD pathology in the elderly population. Early studies suggest that ¹¹C-PiB amyloid PET is predictive for progression of MCI to AD. Further investigation and confirmation of these findings with the ¹⁸F-labeled agents are needed.

15.5 Other Clinical Applications and Radiopharmaceuticals

15.5.1 Amyloid Imaging of the Heart

Involvement of the heart with amyloidosis may be part of a systemic process or localized. Regardless, deposition of amyloid protein in the heart can be serious resulting in heart failure or arrhythmias. Echocardiogram is used to evaluate heart function, and the extent and location of amyloid infiltration can be visualized with gadolinium-enhanced magnetic resonance imaging (i.e. late enhancement on T1-weighted images). However, both of these methods are nonspecific and treatment options may vary depending on amyloid subtype.

Investigations evaluating Aβ amyloid PET imaging for cardiac applications are beginning and promising. ¹¹C-PiB uptake has been visualized in amyloid deposits in the heart in patients with systemic disease and was significantly higher compared to normal controls. Further investigations of ¹¹C-PiB as well as the ¹⁸F-labeled are being undertaken.

A number of additional radiopharmaceuticals, besides those targeting Aβ amyloid, have been investigated for cardiac amyloid imaging. These tracers can be broadly categorized as nonspecific or specific for amyloid or other components of amyloid depositions and are listed in Table 15.1. In general, limited clinical utility has been found due to insufficient sensitivity and specificity.

15.5.2 Imaging of Systemic Amyloidosis

Several of the radiotracers listed in Table 15.1 have been shown to accumulate in extra-cardiac organ infiltration in patients with systemic amyloidosis. In addition, there are multiple case reports of FDG accumulation in amyloidosis.

Further Reading

Antoni G, Lubberink M, Estrada S, Axelsson J, Carlson K, Lindsjö L, Kero T, Långström B, Granstam SO, Rosengren S, Vedin O, Wassberg C, Wikström G, Westermark P, Sörensen J. In vivo visualization of amyloid deposits in the heart with 11C-PIB and PET. *J Nucl Med.* 2013;54(2):213–20.

Chen W, Dilsizian V. Molecular imaging of amyloidosis: will the heart be the next target after the brain? *Curr Cardiol Rep.* 2012;14:226–33.

(a)

(b)

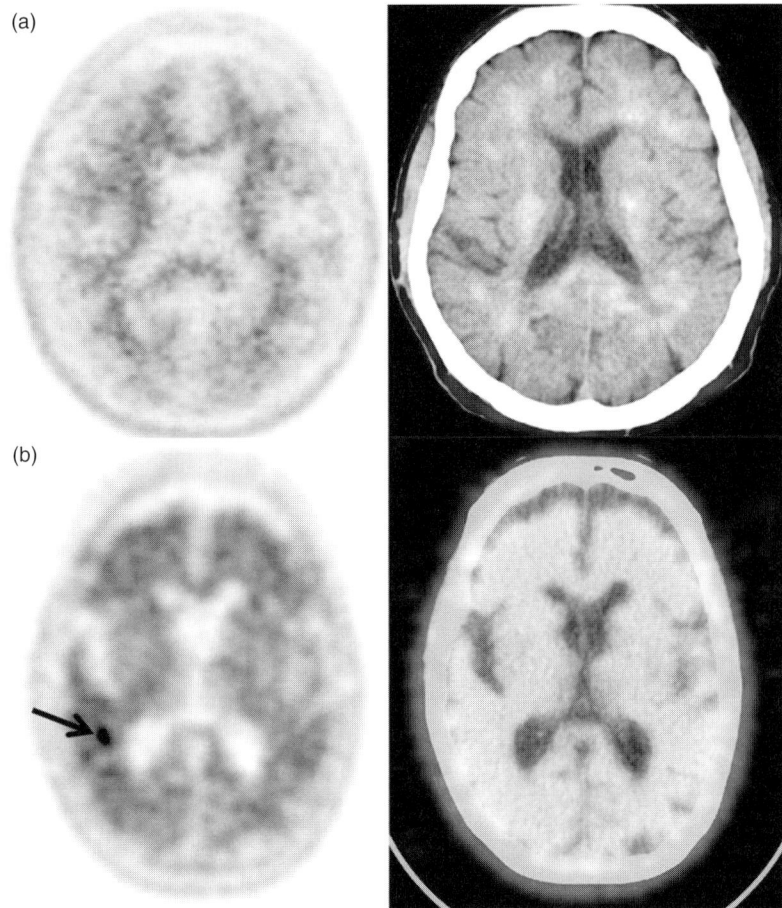

Figure 15.3 (A) Normal ¹⁸F-florbetapir PET Images with normal uptake in the white matter and clear gray–white distinction. Courtesy of Kent Friedman, MD. **(B) Abnormal** ¹⁸F-florbetapir PET Images with extension of uptake into the gray matter, loss of gray–white distinction and focal uptake greater than white matter in the right temporal lobe (arrow). Courtesy of J. Anthony Parker, MD.

Clark CM, Schneider JA, Bedell BJ, Beach TG, Bilker WB, Mintun MA, Pontecorvo MJ, Hefti F, Carpenter AP, Flitter ML, Krautkramer MJ, Kung HF, Coleman RE, Doraiswamy PM, Fleisher AS, Sabbagh MN, Sadowsky CH, Reiman EP, Zehntner SP, Skovronsky DM. AV45-A07 study group. Use of florbetapir-PET for imaging beta-amyloid pathology. *JAMA*. 2011;305(3):275–83.

Drzezga A, Grimmer T, Henriksen G, Stangier I, Perneczky R, Diehl-Schmid J, Mathis CA, Klunk WE, Price J, DeKosky S, Wester HJ, Schwaiger M, Kurz A. Imaging of amyloid plaques and cerebral glucose metabolism in semantic dementia and Alzheimer's disease. *Neuroimage*. 2008;39(2):619–33.

Johnson KA, Minoshima S, Bohnen NI, Donohoe KJ, Foster NL, Herscovitch P, Karlawish JH, Rowe CC, Carrillo MC, Hartley DM, Hedrick S, Pappas V, Thies WH. Appropriate use criteria for amyloid PET: a report of the Amyloid Imaging Task Force,

the Society of Nuclear Medicine and Molecular Imaging, and the Alzheimer's Association. *J Nucl Med*. 2013;54(3):476–90.

Klunk WE, Engler H, Nordberg A, Wang Y, Blomqvist G, Holt DP, Bergström M, Savitcheva I, Huang GF, Estrada S, Ausén B, Debnath ML, Barletta J, Price JC, Sandell J, Lopresti BJ, Wall A, Koivisto P, Antoni G, Mathis CA, Långström B. Imaging brain amyloid in Alzheimer's disease with Pittsburgh Compound-B. *Ann Neurol*. 2004;55(3):306–19.

Okello A, Koivunen J, Edison P, Archer HA, Turkheimer FE, Någren K, Bullock R, Walker Z, Kennedy A, Fox NC, Rossor MN, Rinne JO, Brooks DJ. Conversion of amyloid positive and negative MCI to AD over 3 years: an 11C PIB PET study. *Neurology*. 2009;73(10):754–60.

Rabinovici GD, Furst AJ, O'Neil JP, Racine CA, Mormino EC, Baker SL, Chetty S, Patel P, Pagliaro TA, Klunk

Table 15.1 Other Radiopharmaceuticals Targeting Amyloid

Radiopharmaceutical	Target	Major imaging findings and limitations
Nonspecific for amyloid		
Bone-seeking agents 99mTc-PYP 99mTc-MDP 99mTc-DPD	High calcium in amyloid	PYP and MDP intense uptake later stages DPD more specific for ATTR vs. AL type All: mild uptake nonspecific and indeterminate
123I-MIBG	Norepinephrine tranporter	Impaired cardiac autonomic nervous system indirect measure of amyloid deposition
111In-antimyosin mAB	Myosin	Myocardial damage from amyloid infiltration
Specific for amyloid		
123I-Amyloid P Component (SAP)	Nonfibrillar glycoprotein SAP (stabilizes amyloid)	Rapid accumulation in affected liver, spleen, kidneys Low counts in heart
99mTc-aprotinin	Low molecular weight polypeptide protease inhibitor in amyloid	Normal uptake liver, spleen, kidneys limits evaluation in these organs. Good for extra-abdominal involvement, including heart, but low cardiac signal limiting
124, 125I-m11-1F4 mAB	κ4 Bence Jones Protein	Reacts with AL amyloid (primary amyloidosis); investigational

Notes: PYP- pyrophosphate; MDP- methylene diphosphonate; DPD-3,3-diphosphono-1,2-propanodicarboxylic acid; MIBG-meta-iodobenzylguanidine; mAB-monoclonal antibody.

WE, Mathis CA, Rosen HJ, Miller BL, Jagust WJ. 11C-PIB PET imaging in Alzheimer disease and frontotemporal lobar degeneration. *Neurology*. 2007;68(15):1205–12.

Rowe CC, Ng S, Ackermann U, Gong SJ, Pike K, Savage G, Cowie TF, Dickinson KL, Maruff P, Darby D, Smith C, Woodward M, Merory J, Tochon-Danguy H, O'Keefe G, Klunk WE, Mathis CA, Price JC, Masters CL, Villemagne VL. Imaging beta-amyloid burden in aging and dementia. *Neurology*. 2007;68(20):1718–25.

Rowe CC, Ellis KA, Rimajova M, Bourgeat P, Pike KE, Jones G, Fripp J, Tochon-Danguy H, Morandeau L, O'Keefe G, Price R, Raniga P, Robins P, Acosta O, Lenzo N, Szoeke C, Salvado O, Head R, Martins R, Masters CL, Ames D, Villemagne VL. Amyloid imaging results from the Australian Imaging, Biomarkers and Lifestyle (AIBL) study of aging. *Neurobiol Aging*. 2010;31(8):1275–83.

Rowe CC, Villemagne RL. Brain Amyloid Imaging. *J Nucl Med*. 2011;52(11):1733–40.

Svedberg MM, Hall H, Hellström-Lindahl E, Estrada S, Guan Z, Nordberg A, Långström B. [(11)C]PIB-amyloid binding and levels of Abeta40 and Abeta42 in postmortem brain tissue from Alzheimer patients. *Neurochem Int*. 2009;54(5–6):347–57.

Villemagne VL, Pike KE, Chételat G, Ellis KA, Mulligan RS, Bourgeat P, Ackermann U, Jones G, Szoeke C, Salvado O, Martins R, O'Keefe G, Mathis CA, Klunk WE, Ames D, Masters CL, Rowe CC. Longitudinal assessment of Aβ and cognition in aging and Alzheimer disease. *Ann Neurol*. 2011;69(1):181–92.

Wong DF, Rosenberg PB, Zhou Y, Kumar A, Raymont V, Ravert HT, Dannals RF, Nandi A, Brašić JR, Ye W, Hilton J, Lyketsos C, Kung HF, Joshi AD, Skovronsky DM, Pontecorvo MJ. In vivo imaging of amyloid deposition in Alzheimer disease using the radioligand 18F-AV-45 (florbetapir [corrected] F 18). *J Nucl Med*. 2010;51(6):913–20.

Index

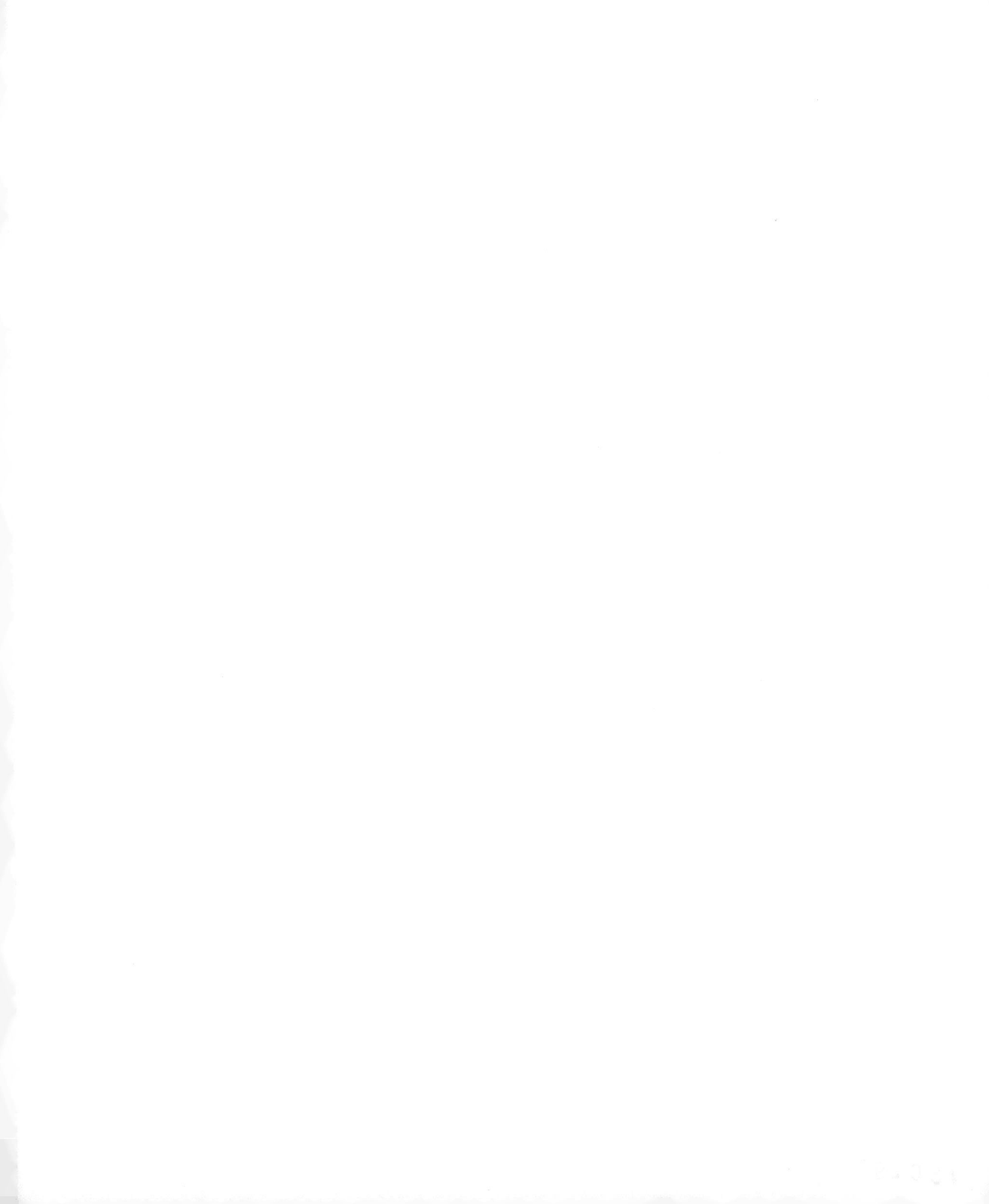